refrep.2006

CL

O G

OXFORD GENERA

Mental

O G P L

OXFORD GENERAL PRACTICE LIBRARY

Mental Health

Professor Tony Kendrick

Professor of Primary Medical Care
Southampton University,
Southampton, UK

Dr Chantal Simon

MRC Research Fellow and General Practitioner
University of Southampton and
Christchurch, UK

and Series Editor

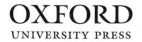

OXFORD
UNIVERSITY PRESS

OXFORD
UNIVERSITY PRESS

Great Clarendon Street, Oxford OX2 6DP

Oxford University Press is a department of the University of Oxford.
It furthers the University's objective of excellence in research, scholarship,
and education by publishing worldwide in

Oxford New York

Auckland Cape Town Dar es Salaam Hong Kong Karachi
Kuala Lumpur Madrid Melbourne Mexico City Nairobi
New Delhi Shanghai Taipei Toronto

With offices in

Argentina Austria Brazil Chile Czech Republic France Greece
Guatemala Hungary Italy Japan Poland Portugal Singapore
South Korea Switzerland Thailand Turkey Ukraine Vietnam

Oxford is a registered trade mark of Oxford University Press
in the UK and in certain other countries

Published in the United States
by Oxford University Press Inc., New York

© Oxford University Press, 2006

British Library Cataloguing in Publication Data

Data available

Library of Congress Cataloging in Publication Data

Data available

Typeset by Newgen Imaging Systems (P) Ltd, Chennai, India
Printed in Italy
on acid-free paper by
Legoprint S.p.A

ISBN 0–19–857057–0   978–0–19–857057–8

10 9 8 7 6 5 4 3 2 1

Contents

Acknowledgements

We would like to thank Jon Birtwistle for his help with this book generally, Dr Francoise van Dorp for reviewing the children's behaviour problems section, Dr Helen Lester for helping us with amendments to the Quality and Outcomes Framework, and Anna Wilson for information and advice on the section on child abuse.

Symbols and abbreviations

⚠	Warning
❶	Important Note
☜	Controversial point
☎	Telephone number
🖫	Website
📖	Cross reference to
±	With or without
↑	Increased/increasing
↓	Decreased/decreasing
→	Leading to
1°	Primary
2°	Secondary
♂	Male
♀	Female
≈	Approximately equal
~	Approximately
%	Percent(age)
≥	Greater than or equal to
≤	Less than or equal to
>	Greater than
<	Less than
C	Cochrane review
G	Guideline from major guideline producing body
N	NICE guidance
R	Randomized controlled trial in major journal
S	Systematic review in major journal
1st	First
A&E	Accident and Emergency
ADHD	Attention deficit hyperactivity disorder
AIDS	Acquired immune deficiency syndrome
AST	Aspartate amino transferase
bd	Twice daily
BMI	Body mass index

BNF	British National Formulary
BP	Blood pressure
Ca^{2+}	Calcium
CBT	Cognitive behaviour therapy
CMV	Cytomegalovirus
CNS	Central nervous system
CO_2	Carbon dioxide
CPN	Community psychiatric nurse
CVA	Stroke
CXR	Chest X-ray
d.	Day(s)
DM	Diabetes mellitus
DN	District nurse
DVLA	Driver and Vehicle Licensing Authority
EBV	Epstein–Barr virus
ECG	Electrocardiograph
e.g.	For example
ESR	Erythrocyte sedimentation rate
etc.	Et cetera
FBC	Full blood count
FH	Family history
GGT	Gamma glutamyl transpeptidase
GI	Gastrointestinal
GMS	General Medical Services
GP	General Practitioner
h.	Hour(s)
HRT	Hormone replacement therapy
HIV	Human immune deficiency virus
HV	Health visitor
IQ	Intelligence quotient
IVF	In vitro fertilization
K^+	Potassium
LFTs	Liver function tests
LGV	Large goods vehicle
MAOI	Monoamine oxidase inhibitor
MCV	Mean cell volume
mg	Milligrams
MI	Myocardial infarct
min.	Minutes

mo.	Month(s)
MS	Multiple sclerosis
MSU	Mid-stream urine
M,C&S	Microscopy, culture and sensitivities
O_2	Oxygen
od	Once daily
p.	Page number
PCO	Primary Care Organization
PCV	Public carriage vehicle
PD	Parkinson's disease
PH	Past history
PMS	Personal Medical Services
prn	As needed
SLE	Systemic lupus erythematosis
SSRI	Selective serotonin reuptake inhibitor
TCA	Tricyclic antidepressant
tds	Three times a day
TFTs	Thyroid function tests
TIA	Transient ischaemic attack
TV	Television
u.	Units
UK	United Kingdom
U&E	Urea and electrolytes
USS	Ultrasound scan
UTI	Urinary tract infection
wk.	Week(s)
y.	Year(s)

Chapter 1

Assessing patients with suspected mental health problems in primary care

1

Child mental health assessment

2%–5% of children are presented by their parents or carers with mental health or behavioural problems as the main complaint, often mixed with physical problems. GPs are often asked to 'sort out' behaviour problems of children by parents at their wits' ends. 2–10% of all children are said to have behaviour problems depending on how the problems are defined and measured.

Differentiation between normal behaviour and behavioural problems can be difficult—especially if you don't know the child or family well. A significant problem is more likely:
- when the behaviour is frequent and chronic
- when >1 problem behaviour occurs, *and*
- if behaviour interferes with social and cognitive functioning.

A feature of child psychiatry is that the child should be seen in the context of a family—any problems are an interaction between child, family and environment. The history is usually taken from the parents but it's helpful if the child can contribute. Older children may prefer to be seen alone.

Assessment: See Figure 1.1

Management: 📖 pp.23–51

GP Notes: Key questions

Important questions to explore from the start:
- Who is most worried about the child?
- Why are they presenting now?
- What do they think should be done about the problem?

Advice for patients: Support groups

Information and support for parents:
Green *Toddler taming: A parents guide to the first four years* (2000) Vermilion ISBN 0091875285
Green *Beyond Toddlerdom: Every Parent's Guide to the 5–10s* (2000) Vermilion ISBN 0091816246
Parentline ☎ 0808 800 2222 🖥 www.parentlineplus.org.uk

Information and support for children:
Childline 24h. confidential counselling service ☎ 0800 1111
🖥 www.childline.org

Figure 1.1 Assessment of childhood mental health problems

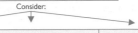

Start by gathering background information:
If the child is present, watch interactions between the child and parent/carer.

It is useful to interview parents both with and without the child and older children both with and without the parent.

Diaries can be helpful.

Consider:

Child
- Is the child acutely unwell?
- Does the child have a chronic illness or disability?
- Does the child have a physical deformity?
- Does the child have any learning difficulty?
- What is the child's normal temperament like?
- Were there any problems in pregnancy or the neonatal period?
- At what age did the child walk and talk?
- Does the child have any feeding or sleeping difficulties?
- Is the child clingy?
- Does the child cry excessively?

Family
- What were the parents' childhoods like?
- Is there family breakdown or marital stress?
- Does either parent or a sibling have a chronic illness or disability? (depression, schizophrenia, cancer etc.)
- What were the circumstances of the child being born? (adoption, IVF, unwanted pregnancy etc)
- Did the mother suffer from postnatal depression?
- Is the child living in care or with short-term foster parents?
- Have there been any major losses e.g. family death or parent leaving?
- What are the parents' expectations of the child?

Environment
- Social deprivation?
- Neighbourhood?
- Frequent relocations?
- How does the child integrate into play group, nursery or school?

Then:

Find out about the behavioural problems
- What does the child do?
- When did it start?
- When and where does that behaviour occur?
- What seems to trigger it?
- How do the parents and other carers/teachers react?

Adult mental health assessment

When assessing a patient with mental health problems in primary care, the objectives are to:
- Establish a constructive relationship with the patient to enable patient and doctor to communicate effectively and serve as the basis for any subsequent therapeutic relationship.
- Assess the patient's emotions and attitudes.
- Determine if the patient has a mental disorder and, if so, which?
- Find out (where possible) what caused the mental disorder
- Establish how it might be treated

Psychiatric history

Informants: Often worries about a patient with a mental disorder are flagged up to a GP by a concerned relative or friend. Talk to the informant (though be careful to maintain confidentiality of the patient), establish the concerns and circumstances and review old notes before seeing the patient.

The consultation: Use open questions at the start becoming directive when necessary—clarify, reflect, facilitate, listen. Be open and ready to ask about suicide, sex, drugs etc. *Ask about:*
- *Occupation*—unemployed? Happy in job?
- *Home situation*—housing, relationships, social support, debt etc.
- *Presenting complaint*—chronological account, past history of similar symptoms. Ask directly about thoughts of suicide and self-harm.
- *Family history*—psychiatric illness, recent loss or serious illness of a family member, bereavement, depression, suicide or attempted suicide, psychosis, alcoholism, drug use
- *Personal history*—abuse (abuse as a child, domestic violence), substance misuse, serious illness (including past psychiatric history and major physical illnesses), recent significant events (e.g. childbirth, house move)
- *Attitudes and beliefs*—How does the patient see him/herself? What does he/she think is wrong? How does he/she think other people view the situation? What does the patient want you to do about it?

Examination: 📖 p.6

Action
- Summarise history back to the patient and give an opportunity for the patient to fill in any gaps.
- Draw up a problem list and outline a management plan with the patient.
- Set a review date.

High risk groups for mental health problems: 📖 p.7

Assessment algorithm: Figure 1.2 📖 p.8

Interview style

Research shows that mental health problems are more likely to be detected where the doctor displays the following behaviours:

- Giving good eye contact from the start
- Clarification of presenting complaints
- Directive questions for physical complaints which might be related to emotional problems
- Moving from open-ended to more closed questions
- Frequently making empathic remarks
- Being sensitive to verbal cues to emotional problems
- Being sensitive to non-verbal cues
- Avoiding reading or making notes (or computer entries)
- Controlling patients' overtalkativeness.

Benefits of listening to the patient: Patients describe a number of ways in which they value being listened to:

- *Connection:* feeling their problems have been understood
- *Reflection:* helping them to clarify or reframe their problems
- *Acceptance:* when others are condemning them
- *Bearing witness:* that they are not alone in their suffering
- *Reassurance:* that treatment is available and can help
- *Ventilation:* to help release pent-up feelings
- *Encouragement:* that they will recover or improve.

5

Mental state examination

Check:

- ***Appearance and behaviour:*** signs of self-neglect or malnutrition, attitude, movements, social interaction
- ***Speech:*** spontaneity, rate, amount, continuity (flight of ideas, loosening of associations—📖 p.19)
- ***Mood:*** depressed or overelated
- ***Thinking:*** form, content, flow, possession—📖 p.19
- ***Perception:*** illusions (📖 p.16), hallucinations (📖 p.18), pseudohallucinations (📖 p.16)
- ***Cognition:*** cognitive screen such as the 6 Cognitive Impairment Test (Table 1.1).
- ***Insight:*** understanding patient has of his/her illness, its effects and need for treatment

Table 1.1 The 6 Cognitive Impairment Test (Kingshill Version 2000)[1]		
Question	**Response**	**Score**
1. *What year is it?*	Correct: 0; Incorrect: 4	
2. *What month is it?*	Correct: 0; Incorrect: 3	
Remember the following address: e.g. John Brown, 42 West Street, Bedford		
3. *What time is it (to the nearest hour)?*	Correct: 0; Incorrect: 3	
4. *Count backwards from 20 to 1*	Correct: 0; 1 error: 2; >1 error: 4	
5. *Months of the year backwards*	Correct: 0; 1 error: 2; >1 error: 4	
6. *Repeat the memory phrase*	Correct: 0; 1 error: 2; 2 errors: 4; 3 errors: 6; 4 errors: 8; All incorrect: 10	
Total		

Instructions on scoring: Ring the appropriate score results for each question; add up the scores to produce a result out of 28.

Score:

0–7	Not significant
8–9	Probably significant, refer, possible dementia
10–28	Significant, refer, likely dementia

1 Reproduced with permission from Dr Patrick Brooke. Further information
🖳 www.kingshill-research.org

Seek out mental health problems in those at greater risk

Women
- More vulnerable to depression and eating disorders
- During pregnancy and in the post-partum period
- When looking after children <5y. old, especially lone parents who also go out to work
- When subjected to domestic violence
- During the menopause

People with long-term physical health problems
- Diabetes
- Heart disease
- Cancers, and terminal illness
- Disabling neurological disorders: stroke, parkinson's disease, multiple sclerosis, motor neurone disease

People suffering adverse life events
- Bereavement
- Divorce
- Unemployment
- Financial problems

Minority ethnic groups: More likely to suffer mental health problems due to social and economic deprivation, isolation from their usual culture, racism, and past exposure to war or torture (>50% of refugees have mental disorders).

Use:
- Simple language and open questions, and give more time
- Interpreters wherever possible (e.g. over telephone)
- Two-way checking of understanding
- Written materials in the correct language if possible

- Do not assume a shared Western view of mental health
- Explore symptoms, labels, and beliefs on an individual basis
- Ask about family and community support
- Explore alternative treatments available in own community

Carers: Carers of people with mental health problems are at increased risk of health and social problems themselves. It is good practice to:
- Identify all carers and mark their records
- Check carers' mental and physical health annually
- Inform carers they are entitled to a needs assessment
- Ask patients if you can share information with their carers
- Inform carers about support groups and carer centers

Residents of care homes and nursing homes: ~50% have depression

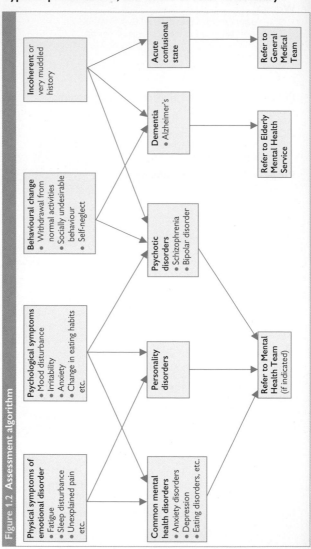

Figure 1.2 Assessment algorithm

Types of presentations, and where to refer if necessary

Physical symptoms of emotional disorder
- Fatigue
- Sleep disturbance
- Unexplained pain etc.

Psychological symptoms
- Mood disturbance
- Irritability
- Anxiety
- Change in eating habits etc.

Behavioural change
- Withdrawal from normal activities
- Socially undesirable behaviour
- Self-neglect

Incoherent or very muddled history

Acute confusional state → Refer to General Medical Team

Dementia
- Alzheimer's → Refer to Elderly Mental Health Service

Psychotic disorders
- Schizophrenia
- Bipolar disorder

Personality disorders

Common mental health disorders
- Anxiety disorders
- Depression
- Eating disorders, etc.

Refer to Mental Health Team (if indicated)

Symptoms of common mental disorders

Non-specific symptoms may be the first presentation of depression or an anxiety disorder. Fatigue, sleep disturbance, and unexplained pain are frequent presentations of underlying depression.

Depression: 📖 pp.56–65

Assessment: Depression is a symptom and not a diagnosis in itself. Assess the significance of depression by systematically seeking out the other symptoms of the syndrome of major depression. This is most easily done using a patient self-complete measure, such as the Patient Health Questionnaire (Table 1.2, opposite). The nine item Patient Health Questionnaire (PHQ-9) depression scale provides an initial diagnosis of major depression and a severity measure which can be repeated to guide treatment decisions. It takes only a few minutes to complete and is an acceptable measure for the quality framework.

Diagnosis of major depression: Major depression is diagnosed if:
- ≥5 of the 9 depressive symptom criteria have been present 'more than half the days' in the past 2 weeks, *and*
- One of the symptoms is loss of interest or depressed mood.

Severity of depression: To measure severity, each of the 9 items in the Patient Health Questionnaire is scored from 0 (not at all) to 3 (nearly every day). PHQ-9 scores:
- 5–9: mild depression
- 10–14: moderate depression
- 15–19: moderately severe depression
- ≥20: severe depression

Management
- *Mild depression:* Patients should be monitored ('watchful waiting').
- *Moderate to severe depression:* Active intervention in the form of antidepressants or referral for cognitive behaviour therapy or other treatment is indicated.

ⓘ *Use your clinical judgement:* for example you may wish to offer treatment even if the score is <10, if patient choice and past history suggest it would be beneficial.

Anxiety: 📖 pp.74–9

Stress: 📖 pp.54–5

Panic attacks and phobias: 📖 pp.80–7

Table 1.2 Patient Health Questionnaire (PHQ-9)

Name:		Date:			
Over the last 2 weeks, how often have you been bothered by any of the following problems? (use "✓" to indicate your answer)		Not at all	Several days	More than half the days	Nearly every day
1.	Little interest or pleasure in doing things	0	1	2	3
2.	Feeling down, depressed, or hopeless	0	1	2	3
3.	Trouble falling or staying asleep, or sleeping too much	0	1	2	3
4.	Feeling tired or having little energy	0	1	2	3
5.	Poor appetite or overeating	0	1	2	3
6.	Feeling bad about yourself, or that you are a failure or have let yourself or your family down	0	1	2	3
7.	Trouble concentrating on things, such as reading the newspaper or watching television	0	1	2	3
8.	Moving or speaking so slowly that other people could have noticed. Or the opposite—being so fidgety or restless that you have been moving around a lot more than usual	0	1	2	3
9.	Thoughts that you would be better off dead, or of hurting yourself in some way	0	1	2	3
	Add columns:				
				Total:	
10.	If you ticked off *any* problems, how *difficult* have these problems made it for you to do your work, take care of things at home, or get along with other people?	Not difficult at all			
		Somewhat difficult			
		Very difficult			
		Extremely difficult			

11

Tired all the time

Fatigue is common. 1:400 sustained episodes of fatigue generate a GP consultation. GPs see 30 patients/y. whose main complaint is fatigue and it may be a secondary symptom in many others. Almost any disease processes can cause tiredness—whether physical or psychological. Physical causes account for ~9% of cases; 75% have symptoms of emotional distress. 2% of consultations with fatigue result in secondary care referral.

Assessment: Figure 1.3

Common organic causes of fatigue in general practice:
- Anaemia
- Infections (EBV, CMV, hepatitis)
- DM
- Hypo- or hyperthyroidism
- Perimenopausal
- Asthma
- Carcinomatosis
- Sleep apnoea.

Management
- Treat organic causes.
- In most no physical cause is found—reassure.
- Explaining the relationship of psychological and emotional factors to fatigue can help patients deal with symptoms.
- If lasts >6–12wk. or symptoms/signs of depression, consider referral for counselling or a trial of antidepressants e.g. sertraline 50mg od.

Refer those with:
- Chronic or disabling fatigue with no identifiable cause
- Suspected sleep apnoea
- Suspected chronic fatigue syndrome
- If referral is requested by the patient.

Figure 1.3 Assessment of patients presenting with fatigue

History:

Onset & duration: short history and abrupt onset suggest post-viral cause or onset of DM, protracted course suggests emotional origin.

Pattern of fatigue: fatigue on exertion which goes away with rest suggests an organic cause whilst fatigue worst in the morning which never goes suggests depression.

Associated symptoms e.g. breathlessness, weight loss or anorexia suggest underlying organic disease. Chronic pain may cause fatigue.

Sleep patterns: early morning wakening and unrefreshing sleep may suggest depression, whilst snoring, pauses of breathing in sleep and sleepiness in the day time suggest sleep apnoea.

Psychiatric history: ask about depression, anxiety, stress; medication. Ask what the patient thinks is wrong and their underlying fears.

Examination: Full examination unless history suggests cause.
❸ Most examinations will be normal.

Investigations:

Suitable initial investigations are: FBC, ESR, TFTs, blood glucose, U&E, LFTs, Ca^{2+}, monospot test, MSU for M,C&S. ❸ Viral titres don't help.

Screening questionnaires for depression can be useful.

Further investigations (e.g. autoimmune profile) may be necessary depending on initial test results, clinical findings and course.

⚠ Don't over-investigate: 1:3 patients have ≥ 1 abnormal result in a standard battery of tests—abnormal results are relevant to symptoms in <1:10 of those patients.

13

Insomnia: From the Latin meaning 'no sleep'. Describes a perception of disturbed or inadequate sleep. ~1:4 of the UK population (♀>♂) are thought to suffer in varying degrees. Prevalence ↑ with age rising to 1:2 amongst the over 65s. It is a serious problem as it can ↓ quality of life; ↓ concentration and memory affecting performance of daytime tasks; cause relationship problems; and ↑risk of accidents. 10% motor accidents are related to tiredness.

Definition of 'a good's night sleep'
- <30min. to fall asleep
- Maintenance of sleep for 6–8h.
- <3 brief awakenings/night
- Feels well rested and refreshed on awakening.

Causes of insomnia: numerous. Common examples include:
- *Minor, self-limiting:* travel, stress, shift work, small children, arousal.
- *Psychological:* ~½ have mental health problems—depression, anxiety, mania, grief, alcoholism.
- *Physical:* drugs (e.g. steroids), pain, pruritus, tinnitus, sweats (e.g. menopause), nocturia, asthma, obstructive sleep apnoea.

Management: Evaluate each case carefully. Many don't have a sleep problem themselves but a relative feels there is a problem, e.g. the retired milkman continuing to wake at 4 a.m. Others have unrealistic expectations, e.g. they need 12h. sleep/d. Reassurance alone may be all that is required.

For genuine problems
- *Eliminate as far as possible any physical problems preventing sleep* e.g. treat asthma or eczema; give long-acting painkillers to last the whole night; consider HRT for sweats, refer if obstructive sleep apnoea is suspected.
- *Treat psychiatric problems* e.g. depression, anxiety
- *Sleep hygiene:* see opposite
- *Relaxation techniques:* Audiotapes (borrow from libraries or buy from pharmacies); relaxation classes (often offered by local recreation centres/adult education centres); many physiotherapists can teach relaxation techniques.
- *Consider drug treatment:* Last resort. Benzodiazepines may be prescribed for insomnia 'only when it is severe, disabling, or subjecting the individual to extreme distress.'

Drug treatment: benzodiazepines (e.g. temazepam), zolpidem, zopiclone and low dose tricyclic antidepressants (e.g. amitriptyline 25–50mg) are all commonly prescribed to be taken at night for patients with insomnia. Only prescribe a few weeks' supply at a time due to potential for dependence and abuse.

Common side-effects: amnesia and daytime somnolence. Most hypnotics do affect daytime performance and may cause falls in the elderly. Warn patients about their effect on driving and operating machinery.

GP Notes: Night sedation

⚠ Beware the temporary resident who has 'forgotten' his/her night sedation.

Advice for patients: Sleep hygiene

Principles of 'sleep hygiene'
- Don't go to bed until you feel sleepy
- Don't stay in bed if you're not asleep
- Avoid daytime naps
- Establish a regular bedtime routine
- Reserve a room for sleep only (if possible). Do not eat, read, work or watch TV in it
- Make sure the bedroom and bed are comfortable, and avoid extremes of noise and temperature
- Avoid caffeine, alcohol and nicotine
- Have a warm bath and warm milky drink at bedtime
- Take regular exercise but avoid late night hard exercise (sex is OK)
- Monitor your sleep with a sleep diary (record both the times you sleep and its quality)
- Rise at the same time every morning regardless of how long you've slept.

Eating problems
Change in appetite
Either increased or decreased appetite can be associated with a wide range of mental and physical disorders. Full history and examination is essential to exclude physical causes and may suggest a psychological cause. Consider depression, anxiety and psychotic illness in all those who present with unexplained weight loss and changes in appetite.

Eating disorders (□ pp.96–9)
Common especially amongst adolescent girls, though incidence is increasing amongst older women too. High risk groups include:
- Young women with low BMI compared with age norms
- Patients consulting with weight concerns who are not overweight
- Women with menstrual disturbances or amenorrhoea
- Patients with GI symptoms
- Patients with symptoms/signs of starvation—sensitivity to cold, constipation, ↓ BP, bradycardia, hypothermia.
- Patients with physical signs of repeated vomiting—pitted teeth ± dental caries, general weakness, cardiac arrythmias, renal damage, ↑ risk of UTI, epileptic fits, ↓ K^+
- Children with poor growth
- Young people with type 1 diabetes and poor treatment adherence.

Abnormal perceptions
Consider:
- **Illusion:** Misinterpretation of visual or other information e.g. a person seeing a shadow of a tree moving in the breeze might interpret it as a person moving. Can happen if the patient has a reduced level of consciousness or occasionally if visual impairment.
- **Pseudohallucination:** Vivid perception which is recognized as not being real, e.g. delirium tremens
- **Depersonalization:** Feeling of being unreal, like an actor playing yourself. Associated with a wide range of mental illness e.g. depression, schizophrenia.
- **Derealization:** Feeling of everything around you being unreal, like in a dream. Often linked to depersonalization.
- **Ideas of reference:** The patient feels he is noticed by everyone around him/stands out from the crowd; media content, e.g. television or radio, refers to himself, or that others are talking or thinking about him. Becomes a delusion of reference (□ p.18) when insight is lost. Associated with depressive states, schizophrenia, and acute and chronic cognitive impairment.

Odd ideas
- **Compulsions:** □ p.88
- **Obsessions:** □ p.19, p.88

GP Notes: Screening questions

Screen high risk patients for eating disorders with simple screening questions:
- Do you worry excessively about your weight?
- Do you think you have an eating problem?

Symptoms suggestive of psychosis

Abnormal beliefs: Decide whether a belief is normal in the context of the patient. If not, decide if the belief is a:
- **Delusion** i.e. a belief that does not seem to have a rational basis and which is not amenable to argument, or
- **Overvalued idea** i.e. belief that is odd but understandable given the patient's background

Delusions: Beliefs held unshakably despite available counter-evidence and which are unexpected in view of circumstances and background. The belief is usually (but not always) false.
- **Primary delusions:** Belief arrives in the head fully formed. e.g. thought insertion; strongly suggestive of schizophrenia.
- **Secondary delusions:** Belief arises on the basis of experience e.g. someone who has lost their job several times through no fault of their own may believe they are unemployable.

Paranoid delusions: Delusions which concern the relationship between the patient and other people. Associated with schizophrenia, depressive states and acute and chronic cognitive impairment. Can be:
- *Delusions of reference:* Ideas of reference, 📖 p.16
- *Delusions of persecution:* Most common type of paranoid delusion. Belief that a person or organization is intentionally harassing or inflicting harm upon the patient. Associated with schizophrenia, depressive states and acute and chronic cognitive impairment
- *Delusions of grandeur:* Beliefs of possessing exaggerated power, importance, knowledge or ability. Associated with manic depression.

Hallucinations: Sensory experiences in the absence of stimuli. May be visual, auditory, gustatory, olfactory or tactile.
- **Visual, tactile and auditory hallucinations** suggest mental illness:
  - Visual and tactile hallucinations suggest organic disorder e.g. dementia, acute confusional state, metabolic encephalopathy, drug abuse.
  - Auditory hallucinations suggest psychosis.
- Hallucinations experienced when the patient is falling asleep (*hypnagogic hallucination*) or waking up (*hypnapompic hallucination*) are features of narcolepsy.
- **Olfactory and gustatory hallucinations:** often occur together. May be suggestive of psychosis but also occur with temporal lobe epilepsy and olfactory bulb tumours.

Thought disorders: Consider disorders of:
Content
- *Ideas of reference:* 📖 p.16

Flow
- *Flight of ideas:* Leaps from idea to idea. There is always some association between ideas but may seem odd e.g. rhymes. Associated with manic illness.

- *Perseveration:* Persistence of a verbal or other behavior beyond what is apparently intended, expected or needed. Associated with dementia and brain damage e.g. cerebral palsy, CVA.
- *Loosening of association:* Series of thoughts appear only distantly (or loosely) related to one another or completely unrelated. Associated with schizophrenia.
- *Thought block:* abrupt and complete interruption in the stream of thought leaving a blank mind. Associated with schizophrenia.

Form:
- *Preoccupation:* The patient thinks about a topic frequently but can terminate the thoughts voluntarily. Common symptom e.g. in anxiety states. Ask about preoccupation with suicide in depressed patients.
- *Obsession:* Thought or image repeated in spite of its inappropriateness or intrusiveness and associated discomfort. The thought and efforts to stop it can be disabling.

Possession:
- *Thought insertion:* Thoughts do not belong to the patient but have been planted there by someone else. One of the 1st rank symptoms of schizophrenia.
- *Thought withdrawal:* Opposite of thought insertion. The patient perceives a thought is missing and has been removed by someone else. A 1st rank symptom of schizophrenia.
- *Thought broadcasting:* The patient believes his thoughts can be heard by other people—either directly or via the newspapers, radio etc. Associated with schizophrenia.

Disturbed behaviour

When a patient becomes very agitated or violent or starts to behave oddly, the GP is usually called—by the patient, relatives or friends or police attending the disturbance.

Assessment

- Before seeing the patient gather as much information as possible from notes, relatives—even neighbours.
- Ask the patient and family for any history of drugs or alcohol excess.
- Listen to the patient and talk calmly—choose your words carefully.
- Try to look for organic causes. This can be difficult in the heat of the moment and physical examination except from a distance may be impossible. Don't put yourself at risk.
- Suspect an organic cause where there are visual hallucinations.
- Discuss and explain your suggested management with the patient and any attendants.
- If the patient is an immediate danger to himself or others, admission is warranted.
- If the cause of the behaviour is unclear, admission for investigation is needed.
- Instigate management of treatable causes identified e.g. admit if MI suspected; treat UTI
- Consider sedation to cover the period before admission or to alleviate symptoms if admission is inappropriate.

Causes of disturbed behaviour
- *Physical illness causing acute confusional state:* infection (e.g. UTI, chest infection); hypoglycaemia; hypoxia; head injury; epilepsy. 📖 p.119.
- *Drugs:* alcohol (or alcohol withdrawal); prescribed drugs (e.g. steroid psychosis); illicit drugs (e.g. amphetamines).
- *Psychiatric illness:* schizophrenia; mania; anxiety/depression; dementia; personality disorder (e.g. attention-seeking; uncontrolled anger).

Acute management: After assessing the problem, decide if hospitali-zation is required and whether this can be done on a voluntary or involuntary basis.

Suitable drugs to use for sedation
- *Oral:* diazepam 5–10mg po or lorazepam 1mg po/s/ling; chlorpromazine 50–100mg po.
- *Intramuscular:* chlorpromazine 50mg; haloperidol 1–3mg.

ⓘ Avoid sedating patients with COPD, epilepsy or if the patient has been taking illicit drugs, barbiturates, or alcohol.

Compulsory admission under the Mental Health Act: 📖 pp.134–7

GP Notes: Violent patients

⚠ Look after your own safety

- If the patient is known to be violent, get back-up from the police before entering the situation.
- Tell someone you are going in and when to expect an 'exit' call. Advise them to call for help if that call is not made.
- Do not put yourself in a vulnerable situation—sit where there is a clear, unimpeded exit route.
- Do not make the patient feel trapped.
- Do not try to restrain the patient.

⚠ **Acute dystonia** can occur soon after giving phenothiazines or butyophenones. *Signs:*

- torticollis
- tongue protrusion
- grimacing
- opisthotonus.

Dystonia can be relieved with im procyclidine 5–10mg (repeated prn after 20min. to a maximum dose of 20mg).

Chapter 2

Diagnosis and management of common childhood mental health problems

Common problems in children

There is no right or wrong way to deal with these problems and the approach outlined here is usually just one way to tackle these problems.

Sleep problems: 📖 pp.30–3

School refusal and truancy: 📖 p.38

Toilet training problems: 📖 pp.28–9

Feeding problems: Parents commonly complain their child is not eating enough or eating the wrong foods. Usually the child continues to grow and develop normally. If so, reassure the parents. Advise them to:
- Restrict snacks between meals
- Show little emotion when putting food in front of the child at meal times and remove the food after 15–20min. without comment about what is or isn't eaten.

> ⚠ If the child is not growing or developing normally, seek an organic cause. Refer to paediatrics.

Fears and phobias

Fears
- Fears of the dark, monsters and spiders are common in 3–4y. olds
- Fears of injury and death are more common in older children.
- Statements made by the parents in anger or jest may be taken literally by preschool children and can be disturbing.
- Frightening stories, films, or TV programmes may be upsetting and intensify fears.

Phobias: cause persistent, unrealistic, yet intense anxiety in reaction to external situations or stimuli.

Management: Normal developmental stage-related fears must be differentiated from true phobias and anxiety states. If the phobia or fear is intense and interferes with the child's activity or if the child does not respond to simple reassurance, refer to child psychiatry.

Tics: Sudden, repetitive co-ordinated movements of no apparent purpose. Commonly involve facial grimacing, head movements or shoulder movements. Average age of onset ≈2y. Tics are present at some point in ~4% of children. Often a family history is present. The majority are precipitated by stress and disappear spontaneously, though some persist into adulthood.

Gilles de la Tourette syndrome: ♂:♀≈3:1. Characterized by multiple motor tics and irrepressible verbal outbursts—sometimes obscene. There may also be repetitive blinking, nodding, gesturing, echoing of speech and/or stuttering. Usually begins in childhood. Associated with obsessive-compulsive disorder and ADHD. Probable genetic aetiology.

Management: Refer for confirmation of diagnosis and specialist management. Spontaneous remissions do occur. Haloperidol or clonidine may help those severely affected with tics. Treat any associated obsessive-compulsive disorder (📖 pp.88–9) or ADHD (📖 p.40).

GP Notes: Simple behaviour management techniques

For simple problems, parental education, reassurance, and a few specific suggestions tailored to the problem are often sufficient. Follow-up is important to ensure that the problem is resolving. If simple measures are not succeeding within 3–4mo., consider referral to other agencies e.g. health visitor, school nurse, child psychiatrist etc. Specific behavioural techniques include:

Behaviour modification: Behaviour modification is a learning process that requires caregivers to set consistent rules and limits. Parents should try to minimize anger when enforcing rules and increase positive contact with the child.

Discipline: Ineffective discipline may result in inappropriate behaviour. Scolding or physical punishment may briefly control a child's behaviour if used sparingly but may reduce the child's sense of security and self-esteem. Threats to leave or send the child away are damaging. *Options:*
- *Positive reinforcement for appropriate behaviour:* This is a powerful tool for controlling a child's behaviour with no adverse effects.
- *Time-out procedure:* The child must sit alone in a dull place for a brief period. Time-outs are a learning process for the child and are best used for controlling a single inappropriate behaviour or a few at one time.

Breaking vicious circle patterns: The child's behaviour (be it normal for that developmental stage or abnormal) evokes a response in the parent or carer which provokes the child to behave in that manner further—thus generating another response from the parent. Try to identify vicious circle patterns and suggest alternative parental responses which make the behaviour futile.

Conduct disorders: Poor behaviour e.g. aggression, destructive tendencies and antisocial behaviour are common complaints. Tolerance varies from family to family. Try simple strategies such as rewarding good behaviour and ignoring poor behaviour ± 'time-out' strategies (□ p.25). If not succeeding, refer to child psychiatry.

Rhythmic behaviour: Head rocking or banging, thumb sucking, self-stimulation, baby behaviour and many other variants all occur during normal development. They usually appear if the child is tired, uncertain or anxious. Reassure parents. Most resolve spontaneously.

Excessive crying in babies: Babies vary in the amount they cry and ease with which they are soothed. Likewise parents vary in their ability to tolerate a crying baby. Babies cry for many reasons—discomfort, hunger, loneliness, separation, boredom etc. If crying excessively:
- Take a history from the parent(s). When does the baby cry? Can he be consoled? What do the parents do when the baby cries?
- Examine fully from head to toe to exclude causes of discomfort e.g. nappy rash, otitis media, eczema etc.
- Check the baby is growing along his centile line.
- Consider family stress (including postnatal depression, □ pp.62–3) as a reason why the parents cannot tolerate the crying.
- Treat any underlying cause found and support the family. Information about behavioural techniques used to manage babies that cry excessively is available from Cry-sis ☎ 08451 228 669 🖳 www.cry-sis.org.uk

Childhood depression: Response to childhood stress e.g. bereavement. Distinguish from depressive symptoms occurring as part of another emotional or a conduct disorder. Most common in adolescence (♀ > ♂).

Diagnosis: Difficult, especially among adolescents. Unhappiness in the teenage years is common (up to 50% of 14y. olds feel miserable; 25% are self-deprecatory and 8% have suicidal thoughts) and does not necessarily indicate depression. On the other hand, adolescents often don't communicate well with their parents and have little independent contact with health professionals—resulting in late diagnosis. *Presenting features:*
- Unhappiness and/or tearfulness, apathy, boredom and loss of ability to enjoy life
- Antisocial behaviour (♂ > ♀) especially after bereavement
- ↓ school performance—may admit to poor concentration
- Frequent unexplained illness or undue worries about health/minor illness
- Self-harm
- Bipolar depressive disorder is not seen before puberty
- Separation anxiety reappearing in adolescence

Management: Unless a mild episode, related to a single precipitating event and no other risk factors for depression, refer for specialist advice. Specialist treatment includes counselling, family therapy, CBT and drug therapy (❶ With the exception of fluoxetine, risks of treatment with SSRIs outweigh benefits in children).

Further information:

NICE: Depression in children and young people: Identification and management in primary, community and secondary care (2005). 🖳 http://www.nice.org.uk

Parenting Notes: Crying baby? Guide to coping

Is baby hungry or thirsty? Offer breastfeed, bottlefeed or drink from spoon or bottle

Is baby uncomfortable, in pain or generally cranky?

- Check for illness or nappy/clothing rashes—check with GP or Health Visitor if unsure
- Talk to your baby and play with him/her
- Change baby's nappy—let baby kick nappy free
- Check baby's temperature by feeling tummy—adjust clothing
- Offer the breast, bottle or dummy
- Offer cool boiled water, an infant colic remedy e.g. Infacol
- Try gentle massaging of baby's tummy or a warm bath
- Try changing baby's position, picking baby up and walking about with him/her or gently rocking up and down or making a soothing noise. Baby slings, rockers and bouncers can help—always follow manufacturer's instructions on use.
- Take baby out in the pram or car. Consider visiting a friend

Is baby tired but fighting sleep?

- Offer breast, bottle, dummy
- Try rocking baby horizontally in your arms or in the pram/pushchair, or take the baby for a car ride or pram walk
- Try a quieter room, softer light or darker room
- Leave baby to cry for a short time
- Use a baby soother cassette or sing to your baby; some very quiet background noises may soothe baby e.g. ticking clocks, or make cassettes of vacuum cleaners, hairdryer noises, etc.
- Check baby is comfortable and that he/she is not too hot or cold—check tummy to gauge temperature.
- Let baby sleep in fresh air
- Try a warm bath

Sensitive baby?

- Handle and talk to baby gently and quietly but don't overwhelm with stimulation
- Try a quieter environment.
- Try to keep to a routine and limit the number of visitors

Still crying?

- Put baby down, shut door, walk out of room for a break
- Give baby to someone else for a few hours if possible. Use any time away from baby to look after yourself, eat well and unwind
- Go out with baby
- Phone a friend or relative, the CRY-SIS helpline, health visitor or GP if unable to cope or worried
- Alternative therapies e.g. homeopathy or cranial osteopathy may be helpful in some cases but always go to a registered and insured practitioner

Toilet training problems

Most children can do without nappies by day from 2–3y. and by night from 2–5y.

Nocturnal enuresis or bedwetting: Affects 30% of children aged 4y.; 10% at 6y.; 3% at 12y. and 1% at 18y. ♂>♀. Tends to run in families.

Causes and management
Physical abnormality
- 1–2% presenting with enuresis have an underlying physical abnormality—usually UTI.
- Rare causes—congenital anomalies, sacral nerve disorders, DM, diabetes insipidus, pelvic mass.
- In all children presenting with enuresis, exclude physical causes with history, examination and urinalysis for glucose, protein and M,C &S.
- If a physical cause is found, treat the cause.

Delay in maturation
- By far the most common cause of bedwetting.
- *Management:*
  - <6y.—no need for treatment—most will resolve spontaneously.
  - ≥ 6y.—refer to the school nurse who can provide equipment and training to control bed-wetting. Techniques used—Table 2.1.

Emotional distress
- Enuresis is occasionally caused by emotional distress.
- The child may have been dry then start wetting the bed at night again.
- If suspected ask gently about any problems the child is having and manage those problems before treating the enuresis per se.

Encopresis: Most children are continent of faeces by 2½ –3y. Faecal soiling after this age usually occurs during the day. *If:*
- The child has bowel control but passes stool in unacceptable places, cause is usually emotional. Expert help from child psychiatry is needed—refer.
- Firm stool is passed occasionally in the toilet but usually in the pants, developmental delay (mental or social) is likely. Try a firm, consistent training programme similar to motivational counselling for enuresis (Table 2.1).
- Soft stool oozes out causing the child to constantly soil himself and smell of faeces, consider overflow incontinence 2° to chronic constipation. Treat constipation. Refer to paediatrics if not settling.

Table 2.1 Methods of enuresis control

Method	Features
Motivational counselling	Child avoids drinks for 2–3h. before bed; urinates before going to bed; records wet and dry nights and changes clothing and bedding when wet. Rewards (e.g. star chart) are given for dry nights.
	The child is reassured throughout that the problem is not his fault and just a developmental problem likely to resolve in time.
Enuresis alarms	An alarm is triggered when the child starts to pass urine.
	In the first few weeks, the child wakes after complete emptying of the bladder; in the next few weeks partial inhibition usually occurs; eventually the child wakes up in response to bladder contractions before he wets the bed. ~70% effective. Relapse occurs in 10–15%.
	The alarm should be used for at least 3wk. after the last bed-wetting episode.
Desmopressin	Synthetic version of antidiuretic hormone.
	Taken at night as nasal spray or tablet.
	Adverse effects include headache, nausea, nasal congestion, nosebleed, sore throat, cough, flushing, and mild abdominal cramps.
	Effective in the short term (for 4–6wk.) e.g. to cover holidays.

29

Parenting Notes: General rules for toilet training

- *Wait until your child is ready:* this usually means when he can indicate to you that he is going to the toilet and has shown an interest in using the toilet/potty. It is helpful to have a potty or child's toilet seat to put on the normal toilet for him to become familiar with before starting toilet training.
- *Pick a good time:* when your child can have a few days at home without nappies in an environment where accidents don't matter. Make sure plenty of spare clothes are available.
- *Keep the potty handy or stay within easy reach of the toilet.* When your child says he wishes to go, sit him immediately on the toilet. Reward any result with praise and don't punish your child for any accidents—ask him to help clear up any mess and re-inforce that it would be better to use the potty/toilet next time.
- *Until both you and your child are confident in your child's ability to use the toilet continue using nappies when out and at night.* Take your child to the toilet at night before bed time. When dry nappies are consistently noted in the mornings, try without nappies at night—a plastic sheet on the mattress is a good idea. Even when your child has been dry day and night for some time, accidents are common if your child is tired, unwell or unsettled—whether excited or unhappy.

🄳 If your child does not succeed within a few days, either try training pants or revert to nappies and try again at a later date.

Information for parents of children with enuresis:

ERIC (enuresis resource and information) 🖳 www.eric.org.uk

Childhood sleep problems

Sleeping patterns and habits of children vary considerably and should only be regarded as problems when they are presented as such by the family. First take a careful history. Ask about:
- **Medical problems** e.g. night cough related to asthma, itching from eczema, obstructive sleep apnoea. Treat appropriately.
- **Physical problems** e.g. hunger or cold
- **Night terrors** (📖 p.32)
- **The sleep pattern**—usually ≥1 of:
  - Difficulty settling
  - Waking during the night
  - Waking early in the morning
- **The amount of daytime sleep.**

General advice: In all cases it is helpful to recommend a regular calming bedtime routine (e.g. bath, story, cuddle, bed) and minimal fuss when a child does wake at night e.g. try to settle back to sleep without taking out of cot, not rewarding waking with games, snacks etc.

Resistance to going to bed: The baby/child who cries incessantly when put to bed is a common problem with a peak age of 1–2y. The child cries when left alone or climbs out of bed and seeks the parents.
Causes include:
- Separation anxiety
- Increasing attempts by the child to control his environment
- Long naps late in the afternoon
- Rough, overstimulating play before bedtime
- A disturbed parent-child relationship and/or tension in the home.

Management: Letting the child stay up, staying in the room and comforting the child or punishing the child are all ineffective. Options include:
- *Leaving the child to cry:* this often does work and the crying diminishes after a few nights but it is very hard for parents to do and can be impossible if they are in shared accommodation.
- *Controlled crying:* the child is left to cry for a set length of time e.g. 2–10min. before the parent returns to settle him again with minimum fuss and then leaves. Length of time before returning is gradually ↑. Easier for parents than leaving the child to cry and still effective.
- *Staying with the child until he sleeps but gradually withdrawing proximity* e.g. sit on bed with child, after a few nights sit next to bed, then nearer door etc. until child learns to go to sleep alone, this method is gentler than the above but may take longer.

Parenting Notes: Checklist for settling babies (0–6 months)

- Try to put baby down awake allowing him to settle down himself. Do not go back at the first whimper. It is worth noting that young babies often need to cry for a period to get themselves to sleep.
- Young babies will often wake for a night feed; this is natural. However, try to keep feeds as low key as possible (no eye contact, no loud noises, subdued lighting). This will help baby distinguish between day and night and will hopefully prevent night feeds from becoming a comfortable habit as s/he gets older.
- Make sure that baby is comfortable (check nappy), well fed and not thirsty.
- Is baby cold or in a draught?
- Is baby too hot? It is very important not to allow baby to get overheated.
- Some babies like dark, others a soft nightlight.
- Some babies like background noise. Various soother tapes are widely available and may help baby to fall asleep. Try the static noise from the radio which can have a soothing effect. Ordinary household appliances often work in this way too (vacuum cleaner, hairdryer etc.). Sudden noises should be avoided.
- Music can often help babies to settle; try a mobile or musical cot toy
- Rhythmic movement often calms babies. The motion of a pram or motorized crib or a swinging seat can have an hypnotic effect. Baby slings provide continual movement with the additional comfort of closeness with Mum or Dad.
- Playthings on the cot can prevent boredom and make the cot a more enjoyable place to be, especially as baby gets to 3 months or older. Soft toys in the cot can act as insulation—avoid overheating baby.

Checklist for settling older babies and young children (7 months—3 years)—📖 p.33

Information and support for parents:
Parentline ☎ 0808 800 2222 🖥 www.parentlineplus.org.uk
Cry-sis Support for families with crying and sleepless babies
☎ 08451 228 669 🖥 www.cry-sis.org.uk

31

Waking during the night: Occurs in 50% children aged 6–12mo. and is related to separation anxiety. In older children, episodes often follow a stressful event (e.g. moving, illness).

Management: Allowing the child to sleep with the parents, playing, feeding, or punishing the child usually prolongs the problem.
- Try the methods used for resistance to going to bed (opposite)—but advise parents to always check to see that the child is not ill/needing a clean nappy etc before being left to cry.
- Scheduled waking where a child is woken 15–60mins before the time he usually wakes and then resettled has also been shown to improve night waking.
- If a child wakes early, another strategy is to make toys or books accessible. The child may then amuse himself for a period of time without disturbing his parents. Some 2–3y. olds wander around without waking the parents—fitting a stair gate across the child's bedroom door prevents the child coming to any harm doing this.
- Use of sedatives e.g. alimemazine (for children >2y.) is often discouraged but can be useful particularly when parents feel desperate. Only use as a short-term measure.

Nightmares: Occur during rapid eye movement (REM) sleep. Nightmares can be caused by frightening experiences (e.g. scary stories, television violence), particularly in 3–4y. olds. The child usually becomes fully awake and can vividly recall the details of the nightmare. An occasional nightmare is normal, but persistent or frequent nightmares warrant evaluation by an expert.

Sleepwalking (somnambulism): Involves walking clumsily, usually avoiding objects. The child appears confused but not frightened. 15% of children age 5–12y. have sleepwalked ≥1 time. It is most common amongst school-aged boys and may be triggered by stressful events.
- Advise parents/carers not to try to wake the child.
- If the child is in danger, gently steer him away from any harm.
- If the child sleep walks frequently, consider taking action to prevent the child coming to any harm whilst sleepwalking e.g. stair gate across bedroom door.
- If the sleepwalks occur repeatedly at the same time, waking the child ~15mins. before the predicted time can break the cycle.

Night terror: Sudden awakening with inconsolable panic and screaming. Usually in the first 1–3h. of sleep. Episodes last seconds → minutes.
Features:
- Blank or confused stares
- Incomplete arousal with poor responsiveness to people
- Amnesia for the episode.

Most common in children aged 3–8y. and require no treatment apart from simple reassurance. Advise parents not to wake the child as this ↑ disturbance. If frequent consider waking the child before episodes occur and keeping the child awake for a few minutes to break the cycle. If the terrors persist beyond 8y., consider a diagnosis of temporal lobe epilepsy.

Parenting Notes: Checking routine for older babies and young children (7 months–3 years)

1. Ensure both parents and baby are well. Give yourself 2 clear weeks when you are not going out in the evening or going away.
2. Babies and children need a routine, especially at bedtime. Set a bedtime and stick to it. Make sure there is a good 'winding down' period: quiet games, stories and a relaxing bath.
3. Put baby to bed, tuck him in, say 'good night' and leave. Make sure he has any comfort objects with him before you go.
4. When he cries, leave him for a set time (5–10 minutes) then go back, 'check' him, tuck him in and leave. Do not pick him up. Do this until he goes to sleep; some parents leave the period of time between checking a little longer each time.
5. If your child gets up return him gently but firmly to bed. Ensure he knows you mean business and that you are not going to give in. It may help to use the same repetitive phrase and tone of voice each time you go in to your child.
6. Do not give drinks (unless the weather is exceptionally hot), cuddles or stories as this can be interpreted as a 'reward' for not going to sleep.
7. Be determined. If you give in now he will try much harder the next time; he knows you will give in in the end.
8. If baby wakes in the night do exactly the same as before. Go back as many times as is necessary to 'check'. In this way you and your baby know everything is OK.
9. Be consistent. If you have the support of a partner, make sure you work together.
10. Be prepared for a battle of wills. Baby will not give in without a fight. Tell your neighbours what you are going to do and discuss it with your health visitor.

The Gradual Retreat Method: This method is probably easier on the nerves (less crying) but will take longer than the checking routine. Like the checking routine you will still need a routine but, instead of leaving, you stay and sit by the cot or bed until baby falls asleep—stroking him as necessary. Over the next few nights gradually sit further away from him until he will go to sleep with you outside the bedroom door.

Checklist for settling babies (0–6 months): 📖 p.31

Information and support for parents:
Parentline ☎ 0808 800 2222 🖳 www.parentlineplus.org.uk
Cry-sis Support for families with crying and sleepless babies
☎ 08451 228 669 🖳 www.cry-sis.org.uk

Functional pains in childhood

Recurrent abdominal pain: Occurs in 1:9 children. ♀:♂ ≈ 4:3. Rare before 4–5y. Peak age of presentation is 8–10y. with another peak in girls during early adolescence.

Presentation: The child complaints of recurrent pain—usually colicky in nature. Site and character is variable though it is most commonly central. There are 2 types of recurrent abdominal pain:

- Those due to organic disease (such as coeliac disease or constipation) *and*
- Those due to functional illness (~90%).

Examination

- If possible, examine the abdomen both whilst the child is in pain and between painful episodes.
- Check for palpable masses and organomegaly—both require urgent investigation.
- Any guarding or rebound tenderness suggests an organic cause.
- If the pain is functional, examination will be normal.

Investigation

- If examination is normal and there are no symptoms suggesting organic disease, check MSU for M,C & S and consider a FBC and ESR. Record the weight of the child at the first assessment and recheck at subsequent visits.
- If there are any accompanying symptoms or signs, consider abdominal ± renal USS and/or referral to paediatrics.

Management of functional abdominal pain

- Acknowledge the pain is real and the worries of both parents and child. Reassure them that there is no serious underlying cause like appendicitis.
- Suggest a balanced diet with plenty of roughage. Encourage adequate fluid intake.
- Reserve paracetamol for episodes of more severe pain than is usual.
- Stress that if the pain changes or is unusually severe, the child should be reassessed by a doctor.
- Most children recover spontaneously with time though a proportion develop other recurrent pains and some continue to have pain as adults.

GP Notes: How can I differentiate functional and organic pain?

- The further away the pain is from the umbilicus—the more likely it is to be organic.
- Investigate all children with loin pain to exclude renal causes.
- Accompanying symptoms (e.g. weight ↓, dysuria or ↑ frequency, regular periodicity) also make an organic cause more likely.
- Other behavioural or psychological problems (e.g. school refusal, irrational fears) make a functional diagnosis more likely.

Recurrent headache: Recurrent headache with no obvious cause is common in children and a source of much parental anxiety with parents particularly fearing brain tumours.

Presentation
- Site and character are variable—most commonly frontal.
- Accompanying symptoms (e.g. neurological symptoms, headache worse in the early morning) make an organic cause more likely.
- Increasing severity of headache with time requires investigation.
- Aura preceding the headache may suggest classical migraine
- Other behavioural or psychological problems (e.g. school refusal, irrational fears) make a functional diagnosis more likely.
- Nausea and vomiting may accompany any type of headache.

Examination
- In acute, severe headache, check no fever and examine for photophobia, purpuric skin rash and neck stiffness.
- Neurological examination—including gait, cranial nerves, fundi for papilloedema and visual acuity in both eyes (a young child can lose vision in 1 eye without noticing).
- Neck and face—looking for local tenderness e.g. from a tooth abscess or sinusitis.
- If the pain is functional, examination will be normal.

Investigation
- In young children, measure head circumference and plot on a centile chart.
- Suggest parents have the child's eyes tested (free <16y.).
- No further investigations are needed if the examination is normal and there are no symptoms suggesting organic disease.
- If there are any symptoms suggesting an intracranial cause, refer to paediatrics—as an emergency if neurological signs or papilloedema.

Management of functional headache
- Acknowledge the pain is real and the worries of both parents and child. Reassure them that there is no serious underlying cause like a brain tumour.
- Encourage adequate fluid intake.
- Reserve paracetamol for episodes of more severe pain than usual.
- Stress that if the pain should change or be unusually severe the child should be reassessed by a doctor.
- Most children recover spontaneously with time.

⚠ If, despite reassurance, there is still significant parental worry, refer to paediatrics.

Table 2.3 Differential diagnosis of headache in children

	Cause	Features	Management
Acute new headache	Meningitis	Fever, photophobia, stiff neck, rash, photophobia	IV or IM penicillin V and immediate admission
	Encephalitis	Fever, confusion, ↓ conscious level	Immediate admission
	Subarachnoid haemorrhage	'Thunder-clap' or very sudden onset headache ± stiff neck.	Immediate admission
	Head injury	Bruising/ injury; ↓ conscious level, amnesia	Consider admission
	Acute febrile illness	Features of underlying illness e.g. URTI, tonsillitis	Treat underlying cause
	Sinusitis	Tender over sinuses ± history of URTI.	Treat with steam, analgesia ± antibiotics
	Dental caries	Facial pain ± tenderness	Treat with analgesia ± antibiotics—refer to dentist
	Tropical illness	History of travel, fever	Refer to paediatrics for urgent investigation
Acute recurrent headache	Migraine	Aura, visual disturbance, nausea/ vomiting, triggers.	Treat with analgesia. Consider prophylaxis if frequent or disabling attacks.
	Recurrent functional headache	See p.36 (opposite)	See p.36 opposite
Chronic headache	Medication overuse headache	Rebound headache on stopping analgesics.	Aim to ↓ consumption of analgesics until taken <15d./mo.
	↑ intracranial pressure	Worse on waking/sneezing, neurological signs, ↑BP, ↓ pulse rate.	Same day paediatric assessment

Poor progress at school

~20% of school-age children require special educational services at some point in their schooling. ♂: ♀ ≈ 5:1.

Severe learning difficulty: 📖 p.44

Autistic spectrum disorder: 📖 pp.42–3

Attention deficit hyperactivity disorder (ADHD): 📖 pp.40–1

Specific learning disorders

Speech and language delay: May be a learning disorder, or due to deafness or neurological problems. Usually detected during routine paediatric developmental screening. Refer for hearing assessment and speech and language assessment promptly.

Dyslexia: Affects 3–5% to varying degrees. ♂>♀. Sufferers have difficulties with reading, writing and spelling in their native language. There is considerable overlap with other learning difficulties e.g. dyscalculia and dyspraxia. IQ is often normal/high and the child appears bright and alert. There may be a FH. If suspected liaise with the child's school via the teacher. Formal testing by an educational psychologist confirms diagnosis.

Dyscalculia: Rarer than dyslexia but contains many of the same features. The core problem is a difficulty handling numbers and mathematical concepts. Management is the same as for dyslexia.

Dyspraxia: Affects 2% of the population in varying degrees—70% ♂. IQ is often normal or high. As with dyslexia, children have varying features. Common features include:

- Clumsiness
- Poor posture
- Awkward gait
- Difficulty holding a pen or pencil properly
- Poor short term memory
- Poor body awareness
- Reading and writing difficulties
- Confusion about which hand to use
- Difficulties throwing/catching balls
- Poor sense of direction
- Difficulty hopping, skipping and/or riding a bike
- Slow to learn to dress and feed

Management is as for dyslexia

School refusal and truancy

Children <10y.: Younger children may refuse to go to school or recurrently complain of symptoms (e.g. abdominal pain) that justify staying home. Usually school refusal is a form of separation anxiety, though occasionally it is due to a problem at school e.g. bullying. Advise parents to consult the school—a star chart with a star from the teacher for each morning the child goes to school without a fuss may help. Relapses can occur if the child is absent or after holidays.

Older children: School refusal is a more difficult problem. Speak to parents and child together and separately. Try to ascertain if there is a genuine reason why the child avoids school. Liaise with the school. If not succeeding, refer to child psychiatry.

GP Notes: Questions to ask if a child presents with poor progress at school

- Does the child have a physical illness affecting his school work e.g. asthma, eczema?
- Is the child on any drugs that might affect his academic performance (e.g. anticonvulsants)?
- Is the family stable or is there family upset?
- Does another member of the family have a chronic or life-threatening illness?
- Is the child's home environment conducive to doing his school work?
- Is this school refusal?
- Is the child happy at school?
- Is there a problem with vision or hearing?
- Is the child of normal intelligence?
- Does the child interact socially with adults and other children?
- Have developmental milestones been met?
- Does the child have specific difficulty with certain aspects of his school work e.g. mathematics, reading, writing?

Parenting Notes: Information and support for parents

British dyslexia association ☎ 0118 966 8271
🖳 www.bda-dyslexia.org.uk
Dyspraxia foundation ☎ 01462 454 986
🖳 www.dyspraxiafoundation.org.uk
Children of high intelligence 🖳 www.chi-charity.org.uk
Independent panel for special education advice (IPSEA)
☎ 0800 018 4016 (Scotland—0131 665 4396; Northern Ireland—0232 705654) 🖳 www.ipsea.org.uk

Hyperactivity

Not easily defined because claims a child is hyperactive often reflect the tolerance level of the person complaining. More active children with shorter-than-average attention spans create management problems. Hyperactivity may have an underlying cause (e.g. an emotional disorder, CNS dysfunction, a genetic component), or may be an exaggeration of normal temperament. Often it is stage-related—support until that stage has passed. Simple behaviour management techniques (📖 p.25) may also help. If persistent and associated with learning difficulty or developmental delay refer to child psychiatry.

Attention deficit hyperactivity disorder (ADHD)

- Common neurodevelopmental disorder which interferes with normal social function, learning and development.
- Aetiology is probably multifactorial with overstimulation, family environment and genetic factors all contributing.
- Affects 0.5–1% of the school age population in the UK; rare <7y.; ♂:♀ ≈ 6:1
- ~50% also have disruptive behaviour/conduct disorders, 20–30% a learning disorder and 25–40% an anxiety disorder. Emotional problems, low self-esteem, nocturnal enuresis, depression, family and relationship problems are also common.
- Long-term ADHD is associated with low academic achievement, substance misuse, unemployment, and antisocial tendencies.

Diagnosis: ❶ Many of these behaviours are seen in normal children.
- *Inattention:* Poor attention to detail and organization of tasks; appears not to listen; easily distracted; forgetful; lack of concentration on tasks.
- *Impulsivity:* Lack of social awareness; shouts out answers to questions; difficulty waiting (unable to take turns or wait in a queue); excessive talking—interrupts others; lack of social awareness.
- *Hyperactivity:* Fidgets; inappropriate running, climbing, or leaving seat.

Diagnosis depends on several symptoms being present for ≥6mo. in >1 setting (e.g. school and home) and exclusion of other diagnoses causing similar behavioural pictures.

Differential diagnosis
- Learning disorder
- Hearing problems
- Epilepsy
- Autistic disorder
- Thyroid disease
- Drug ingestion
- Psychological problems (depression, emotional trauma e.g. divorce)

Management: If suspected refer to community paediatrics or child psychiatry. Specialist treatment includes behavioural therapy, dietary manipulation (though evidence is slim) and drug therapy (e.g. ritalin—controlled drug, multiple side-effects, growth must be monitored). Self-help and local support groups can be helpful.

GMS contract		
Learning disability 1	The practice can produce a register of patients diagnosed with learning disability	4 points

GP Notes: Obtaining a school report

Ask the parents to obtain a report from the child's school before referral. This:
- Shows whether the problem occurs in more than one place
- Provides additional information for referral and
- Tests motivation—if the parents don't get a report (or provide a good reason why they haven't got a report), will they keep a child psychiatry appointment?

Parenting Notes: Information and support for parents

Green & Chee *Understanding ADHD* (1997) Vermilion
ISBN 0091817005
National Attention Deficit Disorder Information and Support Service (ADDISS) ☎ 020 8906 9068 🖳 www.addiss.co.uk
e-mail: info@addiss.co.uk
Parentline ☎ 0808 800 2222 🖳 www.parentlineplus.org.uk
Independent panel for special education advice (IPSEA)
☎ 0800 018 4016 (Scotland—0131 665 4396; Northern Ireland—0232 705654) 🖳 www.ipsea.org.uk

Information and support for children:
National Attention Deficit Disorder Information and Support Service (ADDISS) ☎ 020 8906 9068 🖳 www.addiss.co.uk
e-mail: info@addiss.co.uk
Childline 24h. confidential counselling service ☎ 0800 1111
🖳 www.childline.org

Autism and Asperger's syndrome

Autism: A developmental disorder of unknown cause affecting 2/10,000 children. Though autistic spectrum disorders are much commoner (9/1000). $\male : \female \approx 4:1$. Autism is a severely disabling condition for both child and family which requires a great deal of support from the community services including the GP.

Diagnosis: Not apparent at birth. Usually detected from 18mo.–3y. when failure of social interaction and lack of speech becomes apparent. GPs play a vital role in detection and diagnosis.

Screening: Consider using a screening tool such as the Checklist for Autism in Toddlers (CHAT) for all toddlers with problems with social interaction or speech and language delay at the 18mo. check (p.43, opposite). If the 5 key items (shaded) are answered 'NO', the child has a high risk of developing autism. Children failing items A7 and Biv have a medium risk of developing autism.

Features of autism: Triad of:
- Impaired reciprocal social interaction (A symptoms)
- Impaired imagination associated with abnormal verbal and non-verbal communication (B symptoms)
- Restricted repertoires of activities and interests (C symptoms)

Management: There is no proven treatment though behaviour therapy is sometimes tried. Be approachable, willing to listen and prepared to be an advocate for the family if they have any problems. Having a child or living with an adult with autism is very hard. *Advise families:*
- To set unwavering rules for behaviour
- To reward and give more attention to good behaviour
- To contact self-help and support organizations
- To ensure they receive all benefits payable (e.g. Carer's allowance, Disability Living Allowance).

Prognosis
- 70% remain severely handicapped—special schooling is often needed.
- 50% develop useful speech.
- 20% develop fits in adolescence.
- 15% lead an independent life.

Asperger's syndrome (autistic psychopathy): A variety of autism in which a child, from the age of ~2y., shows obsessive pre-occupation with routines and stereotyped behaviour with distress if the environment is altered. Social isolation and linguistic difficulties are absent. Better prognosis than autism.

GMS contract		
Learning disability 1	The practice can produce a register of patients diagnosed with learning disability	4 points

Table 2.3 The Checklist for Autism in Toddlers (CHAT)

To be used by GPs or Health Visitors during the 18mo. Developmental check-up.

Section A: *Ask parent:*

1	Does your child enjoy being swung, bounced on your knee, etc?	yes/no
2	Does your child take an interest in other children?	yes/no
3	Does your child like climbing on things, such as up stairs?	yes/no
4	Does your child enjoy playing peek-a-boo/hide-and-seek?	yes/no
5	Does your child ever PRETEND, for example, to make a cup of tea using a toy cup and teapot, or pretend other things?	yes/no
6	Does your child ever use his/her index finger to point, to ASK for something?	yes/no
7	Does your child ever use his/her index finger to point, to indicate INTEREST in something?	yes/no
8	Can your child play properly with small toys (e.g. cars or bricks) without just mouthing, fiddling or dropping them?	yes/no
9	Does your child ever bring objects over to you (parent) to SHOW you something?	yes/no

Section B: *GP or HV observation:*

i	During the appointment, has the child made eye contact with you?	yes/no
ii	Get child's attention, then point across the room at an interesting object and say 'Oh look! There's a (name of toy!)' Watch child's face. Does the child look across to see what you are pointing at?	yes/no*
iii	Get the child's attention, then give child a miniature toy cup and teapot and say 'Can you make a cup of tea?' Does the child pretend to pour out tea, drink it, etc.?	yes/no**
iv	Say to the child 'Where's the light?', or 'Show me the light'. Does the child point with his/her index finger at the light?	yes/no***
v	Can the child build a tower of bricks? (If so how many? Number of bricks:.............)	yes/no

* To record YES on this item, ensure the child has not simply looked at your hand, but has actually looked at the object you are pointing at.

** If you can elicit an example of pretending in some other game, score a YES on this item.

*** Repeat this with 'Where's the teddy?' or some other unreachable object, if child does not understand the word 'light'. To record YES on this item, the child must have looked up at your face around the time of pointing.

43

Parenting Notes: Information and support for parents and patients

National Autistic Society of the UK (NAS) ☎ 0845 070 4004
🖳 www.autism.org.uk CHAT is reproduced with permission of the National Autistic Society.

Severe learning difficulty (mental handicap)

Arrested or incomplete development of the mind characterized by subnormality of intelligence. May exist alone or with other disabilities. Often noted by a parent first—take any concerns seriously.

Causes: Varied—many are rare. Divide into:

Congenital
- Genetic e.g. Down's syndrome
- Metabolic e.g. congenital hypothyroidism
- Others e.g. prenatal rubella

Acquired: e.g. trauma, meningitis, birth injury

Management: Refer to paediatrics/genetics to ensure no treatable cause is missed. *Then:*

Communicate with carers:
- Explain referrals; test results and their implications; the local system and who is responsible for what.
- Find out about the condition (as far as possible) and tell the carers where to get more information.
- Ensure carers receive information about benefits and housing/schooling options available.

Refer to other community services e.g. paediatrician; district handicap team. Ensure follow up happens and assist with assessment of special needs for schooling, housing and employment purposes. Continue prescription of medication started by other team members.

Manage medical problems not related to disability e.g. sore throats.

Promote compliance with long term therapy ± education or rehabilitation programmes.

Offer family planning, preconceptual counselling and/or antenatal diagnosis for parents of children with severe learning disability and patients with severe learning difficulty reaching reproductive age.

Prognosis:
- *IQ 50–70:* 80% of people with learning disability. Most lead an independent life and require just special attention to their schooling.
- *IQ 35–49*: special schooling, or extra support within mainstream schooling, and supervision may be needed.
- *IQ <35*: severe learning difficulty. Limited social activity and speech may be impaired. Special schooling and medical services are needed. Support and counselling for families involved is important.

GMS contract		
Learning disability 1	The practice can produce a register of patients diagnosed with learning disabilities	4 points

Parenting Notes: Information and support for parents

MENCAP ☎ 0808 808 1111 🖳 www.mencap.org.uk
Independent Panel for Special Education Advice (IPSEA)
☎ 0800 018 4016 (Scotland—0131 665 4396; Northern Ireland—0232 705654) 🖳 www.ipsea.org.uk

Child abuse and neglect

Defined as depriving children of their human rights. These are:
- **Being healthy:** enjoying good physical and mental health and living a healthy lifestyle
- **Staying safe:** being protected from harm and neglect
- **Enjoying and achieving:** developing broad skills for adulthood
- **Making a positive contribution:** to the community and society
- **Economic wellbeing:** overcoming disadvantages to achieve their full potential

Statistics: ~3/100 children are abused each year in the UK; there were 4109 reported offences of cruelty or neglect of children in England and Wales in 2002/3 and every year, ~30,000 children's names are added to the child protection register in England alone.

Presentation

Always have a high index of suspicion. *Suspect abuse if:*
- The child discloses it
- The story is inconsistent with injuries found
- There is late presentation after an injury or lack of concern about the injury by the parent(s)
- Presentation to an unknown doctor
- Accompanying adult is not the parent or guardian
- Sibling has been a victim of abuse
- Reluctance to allow the child to be examined
- Characteristic injuries—look for marks consistent with cigarette burns; scalds (especially if symmetrical or doughnut-shaped on buttocks); finger mark or bite mark bruises; perineal bruising or anogenital injury; linear marks consistent with whipping; buckle or belt marks.
- Multiple injuries or old injuries co-existent with new
- Unlikely sites for injuries e.g. mouth, ears, genitalia, eyes
- Behaviour of the child is suggestive—e.g. withdrawn, 'frozen watchfulness', sexually precocious behaviour, abnormal interaction between child and parents, unwilling to speak about the injury etc.
- Vaginal discharge, sexually transmitted disease or recurrent UTI in any child <14y.
- Failure to thrive, developmental delay and/or behavioural problems: neglect and/or emotional abuse are included in the differential diagnosis of failure to thrive and developmental delay. Any type of abuse may result in behavioural problems.

Risk factors

Parent/carer factors:
- Mental illness
- Substance/alcohol abuse
- Being abused themselves as children or adults
- Ongoing physical illness
- Learning disabilities
- Unemployment/impoverished living conditions

Child factors:
- History of sibling abuse
- Learning, behaviour or physical problems
- Unplanned pregnancy/premature birth
- Poor attachment to parents/carers
- Environment high in criticism
- 'Looked after' children

GP Contract	
Indicator	**Points**
Management	
Individual healthcare professionals have access to information on local procedures relating to Child Protection	1 point
Education	
The practice has undertaken a minimum of 12 significant event reviews in the past 3 years which could include • Child protection cases	Total of 4 points for 12 reviews

Table 2.4 **Classification of child abuse**	
Physical Hitting, shaking, throwing, burning, suffocating, poisoning, including factitious or induced illness	**Emotional** The child is made to feel worthless, afraid, unloved or inadequate (e.g. if developmentally inappropriate expectations are imposed)
Neglect Failure to meet the child's basic needs, allowing the child to be exposed to danger	**Sexual** Forcing/enticing a child to take part in sexual activities—may involve physical contact, or production of pornographic material

ⓘ In practice there is often overlap and >1 type of abuse may co-occur.

GP Notes: How to deal with child protection with confidence

• Make sure you are familiar with the practice and local child protection procedures.
• Make sure you attend child protection training regularly.
• Share your concerns with colleagues and try to use shared documentation and computer templates as much as possible.

Immediate action

> ⚠ Welfare of the child is *paramount.*—not to report abuse is to collude with the abuser.

- Wherever possible, arrange for another health professional to be present during the consultation.
- Take a history from any accompanying adult. If possible also take a history from the child alone too. Do not contaminate evidence by asking leading questions
- Fully examine the child. Ask for an explanation for any injuries noted.
- Keep thorough notes—recording dates and times, history given, injuries noted and any explanation of those injuries.

Further action: Depends on nature of the suspected abuse, suspected abuser (e.g. if someone outside the home is suspected, the child is safe to return home), nature of the injuries and response of the parents. Be familiar with and follow local guidelines and practice policy. *Options are:*

- Hospital admission—protects the child and allows full assessment
- Liaison with social services child protection team (on-call 24h./d.)
- If admission is refused, contact social services to arrange a Place of Safety Order, or the police to take the child into police protection.
- Contact social services if your observations and discussions lead you to feel that this is a child protection issue and follow the referral up in 48hrs with a written referral—you should receive confirmation of your referral within 1 but certainly within 3 working days.
- You can also refer directly to the police particularly if you feel emergency action may be required to protect the child.

Difficult issues for health professionals in child protection

- Confidentiality of medical information
- Sharing information with parents and carers
- Fear of damaging future relationships with the family
- Fear of causing family disruption
- Fear of dealing with other agencies e.g. police and social services
- Fear of being mistaken in one's suspicions
- Fear of missing abuse
- Fear of attending court
- Fear of negative peer review

Further information

DoH 🖳 www.dh.gov.uk
- Working together to safeguard children (1998)
- What to do if you're worried a child is being abused (2003)

RCGP *Carter & Bannon. The role of primary care in the protection of children from abuse and neglect* (2003) 🖳 www.rcgp.org.uk

Department for Education and Skills *Every child matters* (2004) 🖳 www.everychildmatters.gov.uk

Figure 2.1 The 4 step approach to managing child abuse

Step 1	Step 2	Step 3	Step 4
Recognition	**Reporting**	**Enquiry and assessment of risk**	**Intervention**
Health professionals either identify or suspect a situation where a child may be at risk of abuse or neglect.	Suspicions are reported or discussed with social services, police and/or child protection agencies. Concerns regarding a family become 'public'- this is often the threshold at which those in primary care hesitate and step back from the brink.	Concerns and allegations are explored, information is gathered and risk to children determined. A multi-agency approach is usually employed.	Consists of supportive and rehabilitation measures in order to enable child development.

GP Notes: Child protection

⚠ This guidance appears simple—and *is* when abuse is overt—but often it is *difficult* to decide if a child is being abused. If you have worries but cannot justify them sufficiently to invoke child protection procedures:

- Check via social services whether the child is on the 'at risk' register
- Check notes of siblings and other family members to see if there has been any suggestion of abuse in the family before
- Discuss your worries with the health visitor and/or other involved members of the primary health care team.

If any of these sources ↑ your suspicion, you may be justified in investigating further or invoking child protection measures at that point.

If you still are not sure what to do, record your worries and the reasons for them in the child's notes and alert all other involved members of the practice team. Review whenever that child is seen again in the practice.

Mental health problems in adolescence

Changes of adolescence start gradually—from ~11y. for girls and ~13y. for boys—and are complete by the age of ~17y. Adolescence is characterized by rapid physical development and emotional change. Adjusting to these changes causes problems:

- *Concerns about appearance:* Some become very concerned about their appearance. They need reassurance, especially if not growing or maturing as quickly as their friends.
- *Clothes/style* are important to express solidarity with friends and declare independence.
- *Hormonal changes* result in body shape, voice, hair and skin changes, body hair growth and menstruation. All can all be hard to adjust to.
- *Acne* may need treatment—especially if scarring.
- *Dieting and consumption of junk food* are common. Rarely eating disorders develop.

Emotional problems: In the course of their adolescence, >1:5 children think so little of themselves that life does not seem worth living. Emotional disorders are often not recognized, even by family and friends. Over-eating, excessive sleepiness, promiscuity and a persistent over-concern with appearance may be signs of emotional distress. More obviously, phobias and panic attacks appear.

School problems:
- *School refusal*—📖 p.38
- *Truancy:* Usually children who are unhappy at home and frustrated at school. They spend their days with others who feel the same.
- *Poor school work:* Emotional problems e.g. worry about problems at home, often affect school work and make it difficult to concentrate; pressure to do well/pass exams may be counter-productive. Exams are important, but advise parents not to let them dominate life or cause unhappiness.

Abuse: Physical, emotional or sexual abuse may occur in adolescence

Behaviour problems: It is normal for teenagers and their parents to complain about each other's behaviour and disagree frequently. Parents often feel they have lost control over their child. Adolescents resent parental restrictions on their freedom—but still want parental guidance. Advise parents to lay down sensible ground rules and stick to them. Evidence suggests children are at greater risk of getting into trouble if their parents don't know where they are—advise teenagers to let their parents know where they are going and parents to ask.

Sexual problems: >50% of all children will have had sexual intercourse aged <16y. and so fear and risk of pregnancy are part of adolescent life. Those who start to have intercourse early are at greater risk of early pregnancy and health problems such as sexually transmitted disease and cervical cancer. Worries about sexuality for some can add to the pressure. Sensitive support, clear guidance and accurate information is helpful.

Trouble with the law: ♂>♀ Most young people do not break the law—when they do, it usually only happens once. Repeated offending may reflect family culture or may result from unhappiness—always ask about emotional feelings when an adolescent is repeatedly getting into trouble.

Drugs, solvents, and alcohol: Most teenagers never use drugs or inhale solvents, and of those that do, most never get beyond the experimenting stage. Alcohol is the most common drug causing problems for adolescents but consider the possibility of any form of drug use when parents notice serious, sudden changes in behaviour. 📖 pp.106–9

Psychiatric illness: Rarely, changes in behaviour and mood can mark the beginning of more serious psychiatric disorders. Manic depression and schizophrenia, as well as commoner disorders such as anxiety and depression, may emerge during adolescent years. Refer for psychiatric assessment if concerned.

Eating disorders: 📖 pp.96–7

Parenting Notes: Information sources

Information and support for parents
Parentline ☎ 0808 800 2222 🖥 www.parentlineplus.org.uk

Information and support for teenagers
Childline 24h. confidential counselling service ☎ 0800 1111
🖥 www.childline.org
Brook Advisory Service Contraceptive advice and counselling for teenagers. ☎ 0800 0185 023 🖥 www.brook.org.uk
Sexwise For under 19s ☎ 0800 28 29 30

Chapter 3

Diagnosis and management of adult mental health problems

Chronic stress

The word stress derives from the Latin 'stringere' meaning to 'draw tight' and was first used during the seventeenth century to describe hardships or affliction. We all suffer from stress and, most of the time, the pressures of everyday life are a motivating force. A problem only arises when those pressures exceed the individual's ability to cope with them.

Causes of stress: Virtually anything we do can cause stress. The most common causes of stress-related morbidity in the UK are:
- Work problems
- Family problems
- Financial problems
- Legal problems
- Exam stress

The stress epidemic: 105 million working days are lost each year in the UK due to stress (11% of all sickness absence). The Health and Safety Executive estimate that ~½ million people in the UK are experiencing work-related stress at a level they believe is making them ill; up to 5 million people feel 'very' or 'extremely' stressed by their work; and, work-related stress costs society >£4 billion every year.

Presentation: Most patients don't consult their GP with stress unless they feel it is affecting their health. Common symptoms include:
- Mood swings
- Anxiety
- Depression
- Low self-esteem
- Poor concentration and/or memory
- Fatigue and/or lethargy
- Sleep disturbance
- Other aches and pains for which no cause can be found e.g. muscular pains, chest pains
- Poor or ↑ appetite
- ↑ smoking, alcohol and/or caffeine consumption
- Headaches
- Loss of libido
- Menstrual abnormalities
- Dry mouth
- Worsening of pre-existing conditions e.g. irritable bowel syndrome, eczema, asthma, psoriasis, migraine

Management: The GP's role is to:
- Identify that stress is the cause of the presenting symptoms
- Educate the patient about stress and the link between their symptoms and stress
- Try to identify the source of the stress
- Provide the patient with self-management strategies (p.55, opposite)
- Support the patient
- Treat any medical problems arising out of the stress e.g. depression
- Provide certification if the stress is so great that the patient is unable to work ❗ If the stress is work-related, consider putting a statement to that effect on the certificate to allow the employer to take steps to alleviate the stress and facilitate return to work.

Further information

Health and Safety Executive (HSE) 🖳 www.hse.gov.uk/stress

Advice for patients: Chronic stress relief

10 tips for chronic stress relief

- Ensure you get enough sleep and rest—avoid using sleeping tablets to achieve this—see insomnia 📖 pp.14–15.
- Look after yourself and your own health e.g. don't skip meals, sit down to eat, take time out to spend time with family and friends, make time for hobbies and relaxation, do not ignore health worries
- Avoid using nicotine, alcohol, or caffeine as a means of stress relief
- Work off stress with physical exercise—↓ levels of adrenaline released and ↑ release of natural endorphins which → a sense of wellbeing and enhance sleep
- Try relaxation techniques
- Avoid interpersonal conflicts—try to agree more and be more tolerant
- Learn to accept what you can't change
- Learn to say 'no'
- Manage your time better—prioritize and delegate (see below); create time buffers to deal with unexpected overruns and emergencies.
- Try to sort out the cause of the stress e.g. talk to line manager at work, arrange marriage or debt counselling, arrange more child care

Time management made easy: This technique aims to transform an overwhelming volume of work into a series of manageable tasks:

- Make a list of all the things you need to do
- List them in order of genuine importance
- Note whether you really need to do the task, what you need to do personally and what can be delegated to others
- Note a time scale in which each task needs to be done e.g. immediately, within a day, within a week, month etc.

Advice and support for patients

Stress Management Society ☎ 0870 199 3260
🖥 www.stress.org.uk
International Stress Management Association (UK)
☎ 07000 780 430 🖥 www.isma.org.uk

Depression

2.3 million people suffer from depression in UK at any time. 1:5 seeking help in primary care have psychological problems; 1:10 suffer from depression. ♂:♀ ≈ 1:2.

Recognition: ~30–50% cases are not detected, although most of those missed are mild cases, more likely to resolve spontaneously. Diagnosis of mental illness is stigmatizing. Polls show 60% think people with depression would feel too embarrassed to consult their GP. This can lead to 'collusion' between patient and doctor during consultation to avoid any diagnosis of mental health problems, serving interests of doctor and patient but doing little to tackle the problem.

Causes/comorbidity: Associated with:
- *Psychiatric disorders* e.g. anxiety disorders, alcohol abuse, substance abuse, eating disorders
- *Physical disorders* e.g. PD, MS, dementia, endocrine disease (thyroid disorders, Addison's disease), hypercalcaemia, rheumatoid arthritis, SLE, cancer, AIDS and other chronic infections, cardio- and cerebrovascular disease, learning disability.
- *Drugs causing symptoms of depression:* β-blockers, anticonvulsants, Ca^{2+} channel blockers, corticosteroids (though prednisolone sometimes used, especially in terminal care, for the artificial 'high' it can give), oral contraceptives, antipsychotic drugs, drugs used for Parkinson's disease (e.g. levodopa).

Definitions

Major depression: 2 key features: depressed mood and/or ↓ interest or pleasure, which must be disabling to the patient.

Diagnosis: ≥1 key feature and ≥5 symptoms from following list present most of the time for ≥2wk.:

- Change in appetite or weight
- Insomnia or hypersomnia
- Fatigue or loss of energy
- Poor concentration
- Poor appetite or overeating
- Insomnia or hypersomnia
- Low energy or fatigue
- Low self-esteem
- Psychomotor agitation or retardation
- Sense of worthlessness or guilt
- Recurrent thoughts of death or suicide
- Feelings of hopelessness
- Poor concentration or difficulty making decisions

Mild to moderate depression: Some of the above symptoms (but not enough to make diagnosis of major depression) associated with some functional impairment.

Dysthymia: A chronic form of minor depression. Depressed mood for *most* of the day, for more days than not, for ≥2y. *and* the presence of ≥2 of the above symptoms.

GP contract			
Indicator		**Points**	**Payment Schemes**
Depression 1	% of patients on the coronary heart disease and/or diabetes register for whom case finding for depression has been undertaken in the preceding 15mo. using 2 standard screening questions*	up to 8 points	40–90%
Depression 2	For those patients with a new diagnosis of depression in the previous 12mo. the % of patients with an assessment of severity, using an assessment tool validated for use in primary care, recorded in the patient record at the start of treatment.	up to 25 points	40–90%
Records Indicator 9	For repeat medicines, an indication for the drug can be identified in the records (drugs added since 1.4.2004)	4 points	Minimum standard 80%

Specialized care of patients with depression may be provided by practices as a National enhanced service—🔲 p.170.

Advice for patients: Patient experiences of recognition of their depression

Patients say it is difficult to describe their feelings—it was 'terrifying... I couldn't get across to people how I was feeling'. Unlike a broken leg, outsiders can't directly see depression.

Although some say they are desperate for someone else to notice how bad things are, others want to believe they are stressed or 'run down'.

To get a diagnosis people usually have to 'make the first move' and visit their doctor.

Physical ailments associated with depression (e.g. gastric upsets, sore backs, extreme tiredness), can make it even harder to diagnose.

When the seriousness of their depression is not recognized, people can suffer in silence. Those people are often angry about remaining unheard. They feel that an earlier diagnosis and/or recognition of the severity of their condition could have made a real difference to their lives.

Resisting the diagnosis of depression is partly about the stigma attached to depression, but also about trying to avoid the implications.

Sometimes only a crisis (e.g. suicide attempt, inability to work) makes sufferers seek help.

Information and support for patients
Depression Alliance ☎ 020 7207 3293
🖥 www.depressionalliance.org
Royal College of Psychiatrists: Patient information sheets
🖥 www.rcpsych.ac.uk

Patient experiences on this page are reproduced with permission from the DIPEx Patient experiences of Health and Illness database 🖥 www.dipex.org

* Screening questions for depression:
(1) During the last month, have you often been bothered by feeling down, depressed or hopeless? and (2) During the last month, have you often been bothered by having little interest or pleasure in doing things?

History
- Onset including precipitating events
- Nature of symptoms, severity and effect on life
- Past history of similar symptoms/past psychiatric history
- Current life events—stressors at home and at work
- Family history
- Co-existent medical conditions
- Current medication—prescribed and non-prescribed.

> Sleep disturbance and fatigue have high predictive value for depression and should prompt enquiry about other symptoms.

Cultural considerations: Some cultures have no terms for depression and may present with physical symptoms (somatization) or use less familiar 'cultural specific' terms to describe depressive symptoms e.g. 'sorrow in my heart'.

Examination
- *General appearance:* self-neglect, smell of alcohol, weight ↓
- *Assessment of mood:* looks depressed and/or tired, speech monotone or monosyllabic, avoids eye contact, tearful, anxious or jumpy/fidgety, feeling of distance, poor concentration etc.
- *Psychotic symptoms:* hallucinations, delusions etc.

Assessing severity of depression: Rapid, self-complete pencil and paper questionnaires can help determine severity. Significant depression which is likely to need drug or psychological therapy is suggested by:
- A diagnosis of Major Depressive Disorder, with a total score of ≥10 on the Patient Health Questionnaire PHQ-9 (📖 p.11).
- A depression score of ≥11 on the Hospital Anxiety and Depression Scale (HADS) (available from NFER Nelson 🖥 www.nfer-nelson. co.uk), *or*
- A score of ≥14 or more on the Beck Depression Inventory (BDI) (available from Harcourt Assessment 🖥 www.harcourt-uk.com)

> A fee is payable for the use of the HADS or BDI, but not for the PHQ.

Assessment of suicide risk: Ask about suicidal ideas and plans in a sensitive but probing way. It is a common misconception that asking about suicide can plant the idea into a patient's head and make suicide more likely. Evidence is to the contrary.

Risk factors for suicide	
• ♂>♀	• Past psychiatric history
• Age 40–60 y.	• Recent admission to
• Living alone	psychiatric hospital
• Divorced > widowed > single > married	• History of suicide
• Unemployment	attempt/self harm
• Chronic physical illness	• Alcohol/drug misuse

Management of depression: Table 3.1
Management of threatened suicide: 📖 p.73

Table 3.1 Summary of management of depression

Presentation	Action
Major depression and dysthymia	Antidepressant therapy (📖 p.60, p.61) or CBT (📖 pp.100–1)
Acute milder depression	Education about depression e.g. information leaflets Support, self-help groups and guided self-help Simple problem solving strategies (📖 p.61) or counselling (📖 p100–1) Monitor regularly for development of major depression.
Persistent milder depression	Trial of antidepressants (📖 p.60, p.61)
Milder depression with history of major depression	Consider antidepressants (📖 p.61) Monitor closely

Advice for patients: Patient experiences of having depression

Depression is different from just 'not being happy'—there is no joy, life is black and you can't see a future, or remember being happy. Depression is like 'a black pit' or 'trying to run through treacle.'

People feel cut off from their feelings and from other people—like being 'locked in' and isolated behind Perspex or inside a thick balloon. Adding to the isolation, many avoid friends and family in case they are a 'burden'.

Many become tearful and some cry uncontrollably.

Many describe becoming very sensitive to noise, music, and reacting badly to the 'slightest' remark—just wanting to 'sit in a dark cupboard'.

Many also find it becomes very difficult to concentrate and remember things—'I really couldn't string two sentences together.'

Eating and basic self-care routines such as dressing and applying make-up can seem insurmountable tasks—little details of life (e.g. choosing clothes) can become 'enormous problems you are incapable of dealing with.'

Negative thinking is described as 'things going around in your head, so you don't sleep anymore' and you leap to wrong conclusions, even to the point of paranoia.

People have trouble knowing anything solid about themselves during depression—'your whole self gets put into the mixer and could come out in any old form.'

Many people talk about feeling 'bad' and guilty as if they have done something terrible.

Many people have trouble sleeping, and variously wake up early, can't get out of bed, felt like a 'zombie' and/or 'shattered' during the day.

59

Patient experiences on this page are reproduced with permission from the DIPEx Patient experiences of Health and Illness database 🖳 www.dipex.org

Drug treatment: *BNF 4.3.* Major groups are:
- *Selective serotonin re-uptake inhibitors (SSRIs)* e.g. fluoxetine 20mg od—usually 1st choice as less likely to be discontinued due to side-effects. Cardiovascular safety and lack of drug to drug interaction may be of particular importance when choosing an antidepressant in the elderly. Warn of possible anxiety and agitation and advise patients to stop if significant. GI side-effects including dyspepsia are common. Sexual dysfunction and weight gain may be particularly undesirable in young, active patients and impact on compliance.
- *Tricyclic antidepressants (TCAs)* e.g. lofepramine 70mg od/bd/tds—titrate dose up from low dose until patient feels it is helping, *or* until side-effects intrude[S]. Common side-effects include drowsiness, dry mouth, blurred vision, constipation, urinary retention and sweating.
- *Serotonin and noradrenaline re-uptake inhibitors (SNRIs)* e.g. duloxetine 60mg od, venlafaxine 37.5mg bd. Venlafaxine should not be used in patients with heart disease, electrolyte imbalance or hypertension—monitor BP regularly throughout use.
- *Monoamine oxidase inhibitors (MAOIs)* e.g. phenelzine 15mg tds. MAOIs should not be started until at least 1–2wk. after a tricyclic has been stopped (3 wk. in the case of clomipramine or imipramine). Other antidepressants should not be started for 2 wk. after treatment with MAOIs has been stopped (3 wk. if starting clomipramine or imipramine).

Specific psychological therapies: e.g. CBT (🕮 pp.100–1), behaviour therapy, interpersonal psychotherapy, problem solving therapy. Possible 1st line therapies in mild/moderate depression though excessive waiting lists are a limiting factor. Simple problem solving strategies can be tried in the surgery, see Figure 3.1.

Counselling: 🕮 pp.100–1

Exercise: Beneficial in mild/moderate depression.

St John's wort: May be effective in mild depression[S] but formulations vary widely in potency. Side-effects include dry mouthy, gastrointestinal symptoms, fatigue, dizziness, skin rashes and ↑ sensitivity to sunlight. Interacts with many drugs including antidepressants (especially SSRIs—sweating, shivering, muscle contractions), anticonvulsants (↓ effects), warfarin, oral contraceptives, ciclosporin, digoxin and theophylline.

⚠ Don't use concurrently with prescription antidepressants; discontinue 2wk. prior to surgery due to theoretical risk of interaction with anaesthetic agents.

Referral to psychiatry:
- High suicide risk U
- Psychotic major depression U
- History of bipolar disorder R/S
- Failure or partial response following ≥2 attempts to treat R

U=Urgent; S=Soon; R=Routine

Essential reading

NICE *Management of depression in primary and secondary care* (2004) 🖥 www.nice.org.uk

Drugs and Therpeutics Bulletin *Mild depression in general practice* (2003) 4(8) 60–4

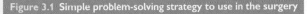

Figure 3.1 Simple problem-solving strategy to use in the surgery

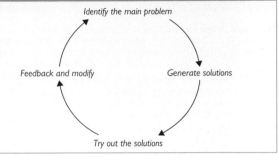

Identify the main problem

Feedback and modify

Generate solutions

Try out the solutions

GP Notes: Frequently asked questions about antidepressants

When should antidepressants be started? Don't prescribe at the first visit as symptoms of depression may improve significantly during 1–3 wks.—'watchful waiting' (*'Don't just do something, sit there!'*).

What should I tell the patient? Giving patients information ↑ compliance. When starting antidepressant drugs explain reasons for prescribing; time-scale of action—unlikely to have any effect for 2wk., effects build up to max. effect at 4–6wk.; and likely side-effects.

How often should I follow-up? Review the patient every 1–2 wk. until stable assessing response, compliance, side-effects and suicidal risk.

How long should antidepressants be continued for? Continue treatment for at least 4mo. after recovery, and at least 6mo. in total. Patients with ≥2 past episodes of major depression should be advised to continue for 2y.[N]

What are discontinuation reactions? These occur once a drug has been used ≥8wk. ↓ risk by tapering dose over ≥4wk. Warn patients about possible discontinuation reactions.

Which discontinuation reactions occur with which drugs?

- *Withdrawal of SSRIs:* headache, nausea, paraesthesia, dizziness and anxiety
- *Withdrawal of other antidepressants (especially MAOIs):* nausea, vomiting, anorexia, headache, 'chills', insomnia, anxiety/panic and restlessness.

Postnatal depression: The law accepts a psychiatric illness is puerperal if it occurs <12 months after childbirth. Depression is a significant cause of maternal death.

At booking
- Take details of any maternal psychiatric disorder, alcohol and substance abuse, severe social problems (including domestic violence) and previous self harm. These are all risk factors for developing depression in the postnatal period.
- When antidepressants are being used for anything more than mild depression, weigh up the pros and cons of discontinuing treatment during pregnancy. There is no evidence treatment with TCAs or SSRIs is harmful to the fetus.

Postnatally
- Be alert to the possibility of postnatal depression in all women.
- Routinely ask about the mother's mood at routine postnatal checks and opportunistically during other encounters in the puerperium.
- Follow up closely all women who have risk factors for postnatal depression.
- If PH of psychiatric disorder, substance abuse or self harm check for signs of postnatal recurrence/exacerbation of the problem.
- The safety of SSRIs in breastfeeding mothers is unclear—older alternatives e.g. amitriptyline are preferable.

Baby blues: Very common—women become tearful and low within the 1st 10d. of delivery. Be supportive. Usually resolves.

Depression:
- Common (10–15% mothers) reaching a peak ~12wk. after delivery—though symptoms are almost always present at 6wk.
- Often mothers do not report symptoms as they feel they have failed if they are miserable after the birth of a baby or they just think they are not coping (and may report that to you).
- Screening questionnaires (e.g. Edinburgh postnatal depression questionnaire) may be useful to detect cases in high risk women.
- Management:
  - Talk through the problems. Refer to health visitor for support[CE]
  - Give information e.g. self-help groups, mother-and-baby groups
  - Consider checking TFTs—especially if presenting with tiredness
  - Consider counselling[CE]
  - Consider antidepressant medication. If breast feeding, tri-cyclics are relatively safe but most manufacturers advise avoiding (BNF Appendix 5). Of the SSRIs, sertraline 50mg od is the safest. In all cases, monitor the baby for unwanted side effects (e.g. drowsiness, respiratory depression). If not breast-feeding, fluoxetine 20mg od is the most effective antidepressant in trials[CE].
  - Refer to the mental health team if these measures are not helping.
  - Risk of recurrence in subsequent pregnancy is 30–50%—women severely affected may benefit from an SSRI through their next pregnancy—seek expert advice.

⚠ Refer to the mental health team immediately if any risk of self-harm, suicide, or harm to the baby.

◆ There is a evidence that oestrogen (but not progesterone) may help some women with postnatal depression[C].

Puerperal psychosis: Much rarer (1:500 births). Suspect if severe depression; high suicidal drive; mania and/or psychotic symptoms. In all cases seek expert help from a psychiatrist. Consider admission—under a Section if necessary.

GP Notes: Risk factors for postnatal depression

- Depression during pregnancy
- Social problems (e.g. poor social support, financial problems)
- Past medical history or family history of depression or postnatal depression
- Alcohol or drug abuse.

Advice for patients: Information and support for patients

Royal College of Psychiatrists: Patient information sheets
🖥 www.rcpsych.ac.uk
National Childbirth Trust (NCT) ☎ 0870 770 3236.
Info line 0870 444 8707 🖥 www.nctpregnancyandbabycare.com

Management of other specific types of depression

Seasonal affective disorder (SAD): 'Winter blues'—recurrent disorder involving 'seasonal' episodes of depression, usually in the winter months. Affects ≈2% adults. ♀:♂ ≈2:1. Peak incidence 3rd decade.

Symptoms: Depression + ↑ sleep, ↑ food intake (with carbohydrate craving) and weight gain. 30% experience elatory mood swings in summer.

Management: SSRIs (particularly sertraline); phototherapy (30–90 mi./d. in early morning—effects should be seen within 3wk.). Light boxes can be borrowed from psychiatry departments, hired or bought (contact SAD Association for more information—🖥 www.sada.org.uk).

Recurrent brief depression (RBD): Recurrent depressive episodes of short duration (2–7d.) which meet criteria for major depression (📖 p.56). High prevalence in primary care. Episodes occur as often as monthly. ≈50% also have seasonal variation. At present there is no effective treatment—antidepressants are ineffective.

Mixed anxiety and depression: Combinations of anxiety and depression are common in general practice—particularly amongst women. Prevalence ~10%. When anxiety and depression occur together symptoms are more severe, there is ↑ functional impairment, the illness is more chronic and persistent and there is a poorer response to any treatment given. Treat as for anxiety and/or depression depending on the predominating features. Refer for psychiatric assessment if management strategies are not working.

Advice for patients: Information and support for patients with SAD

SAD Association ▣ www.sada.org.uk

Post-traumatic stress disorder (PTSD)

Post-traumatic stress disorder (PTSD) is caused by experiencing or witnessing a traumatic event e.g. major accident, fire, assault, military combat. It is estimated 25–30% of those witnessing such events go on to develop PTSD. It can affect people of all ages.

Symptoms: Most develop symptoms immediately after the event though onset of symptoms can be delayed (<15%). However, it is common for sufferers not to present until months or years after onset of symptoms despite the considerable distress caused by them. Symptoms may be misdiagnosed as depression or anxiety. *4 main symptom clusters:*

- *Intrusive recollections*—thoughts; nightmares; flashbacks
- *Avoidant behaviour*—avoidance of people, places, situations or circumstances resembling or associated with the event; refusal to talk or think about the event; excessive rumination about questions which prevent them coming to terms with the event (e.g. Why me? How could it have been prevented?)
- *Hyperarousal*—↑ anxiety and irritability, insomnia, poor concentration, hypervigilance.
- *Numbing of emotions*—lack of ability to experience feelings; feeling detached from other people; giving up previously significant activities; amnesia for significant parts of the event

Nearly $^2/_3$ experience chronic symptoms and there is a strong association with other psychiatric conditions especially depression, anxiety and drug/alcohol abuse and dependence.

Management[N]: Treat any other associated psychiatric illness.
- *Watchful waiting:* Appropriate for patients with mild symptoms which have been present for <4 wk. after the trauma: be supportive and listen. Arrange a follow-up contact within 1 mo.
- *Trauma-focused psychological treatment* (trauma focused cognitive behavioural therapy and/or eye movement desensitization and reprocessing (EMDR): refer (usually via the community mental health team) all patients with severe symptoms <4wk. after the trauma or if ongoing symptoms beyond 4 wk. which affect every day life.
- *Drug treatment:* Should not be used as a routine first-line treatment in preference to a trauma-focused psychological therapy. Reserve for those with continuing symptoms despite trauma-focused psychological therapy or who have refused trauma-focused psychological therapy. Drug treatments include paroxetine, mirtazapine (unlicensed), amitriptyline (consultant initiation only—unlicensed) and phenelzine (consultant initiation only—unlicensed).

ⓘ Debriefing immediately after the traumatic event is unhelpful.

Essential reading
NICE *Post-traumatic stress disorder (PTSD): the management of PTSD in adults and children in primary, secondary and community care* (2005) 🖳 www.nice.org.uk

What type of events trigger PTSD?

A huge variety of events trigger PTSD. These vary from single events e.g. assaults, road accidents, or traumatic childbirth to events which occurred over a period of time or may even be ongoing e.g. war situations, domestic violence or childhood sexual abuse.

How can I recognize PTSD?

- Be alert to the possibility of PTSD when patients present with symptoms associated with it. Ask in a sensitive manner whether or not patients with such symptoms have suffered a traumatic experience (which may have occurred many months or years before) and give specific examples of traumatic events.
- For patients with unexplained physical symptoms who are re-peated attendees to primary care, consider asking whether or not they have experienced a traumatic event and provide specific ex-ample
- Consider asking adults with suspected PTSD specific questions about re-experiencing (including flashbacks and nightmares) or hyperarousal (including an exaggerated startle response or sleep disturbance)
- Questioning children about traumatic events and symptoms of PTSD, as well as parents or guardians, improves recognition of PTSD in children.

Does presentation differ in children? Children, particularly those aged <8 y., may not complain directly of PTSD symptoms, such as re-experiencing or avoidance. Instead they may complain of sleeping problems. All opportunities for identifying PTSD in children should be taken.

Is screening for PTSD helpful? NICE recommends screening using screening questionnaires for those at particularly high risk of developing PTSD e.g. those involved in a major disaster or refugees. In those cases, screening should be organized by the relevant authorities e.g. those responsible for the local disaster plan or refugee centres.

Bereavement, grief and coping with loss

Models of grief

Traditional model: 4 phases to 'recovery':
- *Initial shock:* sense of unreality, detachment, disbelief or 'numbness'. Lasts from hours to days.
- *Yearning:* pangs of grief, episodes of intense pining and a desire to search interspersed with anxiety, guilt and self-reproach.
- *Despair:* The permanence of the loss is realized. Despair and apathy, social withdrawal, poor concentration, pessimism about the future.
- *Recovery:* rebuilding of an identity and purpose in life.

Recent models: Grief is an oscillation between loss and restoration; focused behaviour, demonstrated by swings in mood, thoughts and behaviour between memories of the dead person and 'getting on with life'. Avoidance or denial of loss is common and part of the process.

Health consequences of bereavement

- ↑ *mortality* (heart disease, cirrhosis, suicide, accidents)—particularly in first 6mo. *Risk factors:* ♂>♀, age <65y., lower social class.
- *Mental health problems:* depression, anxiety, ↑ risk of suicide, substance abuse, identification reaction (hyperchondriacal disorder—symptoms mimic those of deceased e.g. chest pain if died from MI), insomnia, self-neglect.
- *Physical problems:* fatigue, aches and pains (e.g headaches, musculoskeletal pain), appetite change, GI symptoms, ↓ immune response (↑ minor infection).
- *Others:* interference with family life, education and employment, social isolation/loneliness, ↓ income.

Bereaved children: Children understand what death is by 8y. and even children of 2–3y. have some understanding of death. Exclusion makes children isolated and often makes the death of someone they have known more, not less, painful. Prepare children for a death if possible and give them a chance to have their questions answered. If a child has problems, seek specialist help.

Abnormal grief reactions: Whether a grief reaction is normal or abnormal depends on individual circumstances—personality, situation surrounding death and cultural expectations. Recognized patterns of abnormal grief are:
- Inhibited grief—grief is absent or minimal
- Delayed grief—late onset *and*
- Prolonged or chronic grief—inability to rebuild life in any way.

If abnormal grief is suspected:
- Monitor carefully
- Consider referral for bereavement counselling e.g. to CRUSE
- Consider clinical depression (📖 p.56) or post-traumatic stress disorder (📖 pp.66–7).
- If symptoms are persistent or worsening despite treatment, or if there is suicidal risk, refer to psychiatry for specialist advice.

GP contract		
Indicator		**Points**
Records indicator 6	There is a system for ensuring relevant team members are informed about patients who have died	1 point

GP Notes: Bereavement concerns

Role of the Primary Care Team
- Develop a practice policy for dealing with bereaved patients[£]
- Flag notes
- Consider staff training and active follow-up of bereaved patients
- If the person who has died is registered with the practice, ensure all medical referrals/appointments are cancelled.

Risk factors for poor outcome after bereavement
Predisposing factors:
- Multiple prior bereavements
- History of mental illness (e.g. depression, anxiety, suicidal attempts or threats)
- Ambivalent or dependent relationship with the deceased
- Low self-esteem
- Being male
- Poor social or family support.

Situations where the circumstances of death may cause particular problems for the bereaved:
- Sudden or unexpected death
- Death of parent when child or adolescent
- Multiple deaths (e.g. disasters)
- Miscarriage, death of baby, child or sibling
- Cohabiting partners, same sex partners, extra-marital relationship
- Death due to AIDS, suicide
- Deaths where those bereaved may be responsible
- Deaths from murder, with high media profile or involving legal proceedings
- Where a postmortem and/or inquest is required.

Advice for patients: Useful contacts

CRUSE ☎ 0870 167 1677 🖳 www.crusebereavementcare.org.uk
Royal College of Psychiatrists information leaflet. Available at 🖳 www.rcpsych.ac.uk
National Association of Widows ☎ 024 7663 4848
🖳 www.widows.uk.net

Suicide and deliberate self-harm (DSH)

🛈 People who have self-harmed should be treated with the same care respect and privacy as any other patient.

Deliberate self-harm (DSH): Deliberate non-fatal act committed in the knowledge that it was potentially harmful and, in the case of drug overdose, that the amount taken was excessive. 90% DSH is due to self-poisoning and it accounts for 20% of admissions to general medical wards—the most frequent reason for admission for young ♀ patients. Paracetamol or aspirin are the most common drugs used. Self-harm is often aimed at changing a situation (e.g. to get a boyfriend back), communication of distress ('cry for help'), a sign of emotional distress, or may be a failed genuine suicide attempt.

Action: GPs are frequently called to patients who have deliberately self-harmed themselves, are threatening suicide or if relatives are worried about suicide risk.

Algorithm for assessment of patients who have deliberately self-harmed, threatened or attempted suicide, see Figure 3.2, 📖 p.72

Algorithm for management of patients who have deliberately self-harmed, threatened or attempted suicide see Figure 3.3, 📖 p.73

Compulsory admission under the Mental Health Act:
📖 pp.134–7

Suicide prevention: *Our Healthier Nation* set a target to ↓ death by suicide by 17% by 2010. GPs play a crucial role in achieving this target. The UK suicide rate is 1:6000 and the average GP will have 10–15 patients who commit suicide during a career in general practice. In ♂ <35y. suicide is now the most common cause of death. The National Suicide Prevention Strategy for England sets out 6 goals and objectives:

- To ↓ risk in key high risk groups
- To promote mental wellbeing in the wider population
- To ↓ availability and lethality of suicide methods
- To improve reporting of suicidal behaviour in the community
- To promote research on suicide and suicide prevention
- To improve monitoring of progress towards the Saving Lives: Our Healthier Nation target to ↓ suicide

Support of those bereaved through suicide: Those bereaved through suicide face special problems. Give as much support as possible, try to ↓ stigma, suggest self-help groups and/or counselling.

Essential reading

NICE *Self-harm: The short-term physical and psychological management and secondary prevention of self-harm in primary and secondary care* (2004) 🖥 www.nice.org.uk

Further information

DoH *National Suicide Prevention Strategy for England* (2002)
🖥 www.dh.gov.uk

GP contract		
Indicator		**Points**
Education Indicator 7	The practice has undertaken a minimum of 12 significant event reviews in the past 3 years which include: • Any suicide • A section under the Mental Health Act	Total of 4 points for 12 significant event reviews

GP Notes: What can GPs do to prevent suicide?

- Early recognition, assessment and treatment of those likely to attempt suicide is key to the GP role—many visit their GP just weeks before suicide.
- Restrict access to lethal agents e.g. avoid tricyclic antidepressants and monitor repeat prescriptions of antidepressants carefully.
- Plan follow-up care for those discharged from psychiatric hospital.

Advice for patients: Information and support for patients and relatives

Self Injury and Related Issues (SIARI) 🖳 www.siari.co.uk
Samaritans 24 h. emotional support via telephone ☎ 08457 909 090
Survivors of Bereavement by Suicide ☎ 0870 241 3337
🖳 www.uk-sobs.org.uk

Figure 3.2 Assessment of patients who have deliberately self-harmed, threatened or attempted suicide

If any self-harm: Assess the situation and admit to A&E as needed

Ask about suicidal ideas and plans: in a sensitive but probing way. It is a common misconception that asking about suicide can plant the idea into a patient's head and make suicide more likely. Evidence is to the contrary.

Ask about present circumstances:
- What problems are making the patient feel this way?
- Does s/he still feel like this?
- Would the act of suicide be aimed to hurt someone in particular?
- What kind of support does the patient have from friends and relatives and formal services (e.g. CPN)?

Assess suicidal risk: Ask patient and any relatives/friends present.
Risk factors:
♂>♀
↑with age
Divorced >widowed>never married >married
Certain professions: vets, pharmacists, farmers, doctors.
Admission or recent discharge from psychiatric hospital.
Social isolation
History of deliberate self-harm (100x ↑risk)
Depression
Alcohol or substance abuse
Personality disorder
Schizophrenia
Serious medical illness (e.g. cancer)

Assess psychiatric state: Features associated with ↑ suicide risk are:
- Presence of suicidal ideation
- Hopelessness -good predictor of subsequent and immediate risk
- Depression
- Agitation
- Early schizophrenia with retained insight -especially young patients who see their ambitions restricted
- Presence of delusions of control, poverty and/or guilt.

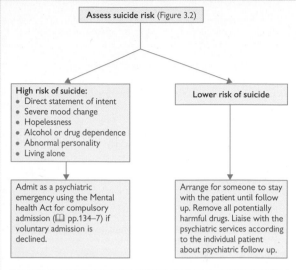

Figure 3.3 Management of patients who have deliberately self-harmed, threatened or attempted suicide

Assess suicide risk (Figure 3.2)

High risk of suicide:
- Direct statement of intent
- Severe mood change
- Hopelessness
- Alcohol or drug dependence
- Abnormal personality
- Living alone

Lower risk of suicide

Admit as a psychiatric emergency using the Mental health Act for compulsory admission (📖 pp.134–7) if voluntary admission is declined.

Arrange for someone to stay with the patient until follow up. Remove all potentially harmful drugs. Liaise with the psychiatric services according to the individual patient about psychiatric follow up.

⚠ **Mothers of young children** who deliberately self-harm or attempt suicide have ↑ risk of child abuse. Assess risks, offer support, arrange for health visitor or social services to visit.

73

GP Notes: Useful questions for assessing suicidal ideas and plans

- Do you feel you have a future?
- Do you feel that life's not worth living?
- Do you ever feel completely hopeless?
- Do you ever feel you'd be better off dead and away from it all?
- Have you ever made any plans to end your life (if drug overdose—have you handled the tablets)?
- Have you ever made an attempt to take your own life?—If so, was there a final act e.g suicide note?
- What prevents you doing it?
- Have you made any arrangements for your affairs after your death?

Generalized anxiety disorder

Anxiety is a normal response to an unusual or stressful event; it is the psychological component of the 'flight or fight' response and is only considered abnormal when:

- It occurs in the absence of a stressful event
- It impairs physical, occupational or social functioning
- It is excessively severe or prolonged

Anxiety disorders are common. At any one time ~5% of adults have an anxiety disorder and ~1:4 will develop an anxiety disorder at some point in their lives.

Diagnosis: Generalized anxiety disorder (GAD) is defined (ICD-10) by symptoms of anxiety present on most days for several consecutive weeks. Two clinical pictures are commonly seen:
- *Acute form:* Sudden onset, usually precipitated by an external event, short course, good prognosis
- *Chronic form:* Fluctuating anxiety over a long period of time.

❶ There is considerable overlap between the anxiety disorders—particularly GAD and agoraphobia, and GAD and panic disorder. Figure 3.4 is a simple algorithm to aid differentiation between generalized anxiety disorder, panic disorder and phobias.

Clinical features of anxiety

Psychological:
- Fearful anticipation
- Irritability
- Sensitivity to noise
- Restlessness
- Poor concentration
- Worrying thoughts
- Insomnia
- Nightmares
- Depression
- Obsessions
- Depersonalization

Physical:
- Dry mouth, difficulty swallowing
- Tremor
- Dizziness, headache
- Parasthesiae
- Tinnitus
- Epigastric discomfort
- Excessive wind, frequent or loose motions
- Chest discomfort/constriction
- Difficulty breathing/hyperventilation
- Palpitations/awareness of missed beats
- Frequency or urgency of micturition
- Erectile dysfunction
- Menstrual problems

Associations

- Anxiety often accompanies depression (📖 pp.56–61) and may be a feature of early schizophrenia.
- Other conditions which can cause anxiety and/or mimic symptoms of anxiety include: drug and alcohol withdrawal; caffeine abuse; thyrotoxicosis; hypoglycaemia; temporal lobe epilepsy; phaeochromocytoma.

❶ Some antidepressants might worsen anxiety and agitation early in the first weeks after treatment begins.

GP contract			
Indicators		**Points**	**Payment Scheme**
Records Indicator 9	For repeat medicines, an indication for the drug can be identified in the records (for drugs added to the repeat prescription with effect from 1 April 2004).	4 points	Minimum standard 80%

Figure 3.4 Differentiation of anxiety disorders

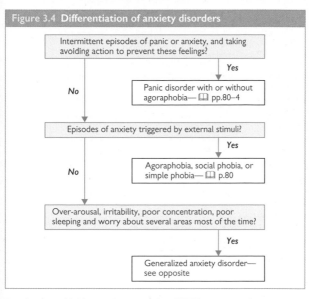

Intermittent episodes of panic or anxiety, and taking avoiding action to prevent these feelings?

Yes → Panic disorder with or without agoraphobia— 📖 pp.80–4

No ↓

Episodes of anxiety triggered by external stimuli?

Yes → Agoraphobia, social phobia, or simple phobia— 📖 p.80

No ↓

Over-arousal, irritability, poor concentration, poor sleeping and worry about several areas most of the time?

Yes → Generalized anxiety disorder— see opposite

Reproduced in modified format with permission from NICE 🖥 www.nice.org.uk

Management

NICE recommends a stepped approach to management of generalized anxiety disorder (Figure 3.5).

Step 1: Recognition and diagnosis

- Be alert to diagnosis—particularly in patients with unexplained physical symptoms who present frequently to primary care.
- Take a chronological account of symptoms and ask the patient's views and beliefs about nature and cause.
- Ask directly about symptoms of anxiety.
- Consider using an anxiety scale (🕮 pp.78–9) to reinforce diagnosis and give a baseline measure of severity.
- Exclude other potential causes of similar symptoms and associated conditions e.g. check TFTs to exclude thyrotoxicosis; ask about caffeine ingestion, substance abuse and alcohol consumption; ask about depression.

Step 2: Primary care management

If immediate management of GAD is necessary, consider:
- Support and information
- Problem-solving (🕮 p.100)
- Benzodiazepines e.g. diazepam 2–5mg tds prn ⚠ Don't use >2–4wk.

In all cases discuss and consider longer term options:

Psychological therapy: refer for CBT (🕮 pp.100–1) ❶ often limited by availability in the community within a reasonable time frame.

Drug treatment: SSRIs e.g. paroxetine are drugs of choice (🕮 p.60).
- Warn patients that transient ↑ in anxiety on starting treatment and GI side-effects are common, and that they are unlikely to see improvements for 2wk. Minimize initial side-effects by starting at low dose and increasing slowly until there is a satisfactory response.
- Review <2wk. after starting treatment and at 4, 6, & 12 wk. If one SSRI is not suitable, or there is no improvement after 12 wk., offer another SSRI/SNRI (if appropriate) or another form of treatment.
- If effective, continue treatment for ≥6mo. reviewing every 8–12wk. Minimize discontinuation symptoms by tapering dose over an extended time period.

Self-help: Options are:
- Bibliotherapy based on CBT principles (🕮 pp.100–1)
- Information about support groups
- Consider large group CBT where available
- Exercise—may benefit health generally
- Computerized CBT (🕮 p.101)

Step 3: Review and offer alternative treatment: Anxiety scales can be useful in monitoring treatment. If treatment is complete and there has been no improvement, consider trying another type of intervention.

Step 4: Reasons to refer to specialist mental health services

- Significant symptoms despite treatment with 2 different interventions (CBT, medication and/or bibliotherapy)

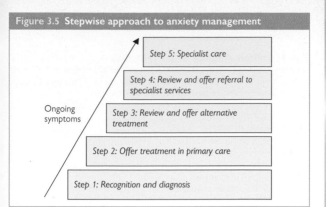

Figure 3.5 Stepwise approach to anxiety management

Step 5: Specialist care

Step 4: Review and offer referral to specialist services

Step 3: Review and offer alternative treatment

Step 2: Offer treatment in primary care

Step 1: Recognition and diagnosis

Ongoing symptoms

GP Notes: Ways of improving outcome

Discuss treatment options: Shared decision-making between the individual and healthcare professionals improves concordance and clinical outcomes.

Provide information: Information in a form suitable to patients and/or carers about the nature, course and treatment of their anxiety disorder—including information on use and likely side-effects of any medication improves concordance and clinical outcomes.

Advice for patients: Information and support for patients

Anxiety Care Helpline ☎ 020 8478 3400 🖳 www.anxietycare.org.uk
No more panic 🖳 www.nomorepanic.co.uk
Royal College of Psychiatrists: Patient information sheets
🖳 www.rcpsych.ac.uk

Essential reading

NICE Management of anxiety (panic disorder, with or without agoraphobia, and generalized anxiety disorder) in adults in primary, secondary and community care (2004) 🖳 www.nice.org.uk

The Hamilton Anxiety Scale (HAMA): is a rating scale developed to quantify severity of anxiety symptoms. It consists of 14 items, each defined by a series of symptoms which the clinician goes through with the patient. Each item is rated on a 5-point scale:

0—not present
1—mild symptoms
2—moderate symptoms
3—severe symptoms
4—incapacitating symptoms

At the end the score is totaled to give a measure of anxiety severity:

- Score 18–24—mild anxiety
- Score 25–29—moderate anxiety
- Score ≥30—severe anxiety

Alternative measures: include

- The Hospital Anxiety and Depression Scale (HADS) (available from NFER Nelson ▢ www.nfer-nelson.co.uk), *or*
- The Beck Anxiety Inventory (BDI) (available from Harcourt Assessment ▢ www.harcourt-uk.com)

🛈 a fee is payable for the use of both these measures. The HAMA can be used free of charge.

Table 3.2 The Hamilton Anxiety Score

Name:	Date:	
Symptom	Description	Score (0–4)
Anxious mood	Worries Anticipates worst	
Tension	Startles Cries easily Restless Trembling	
Fears	Fear of the dark Fear of strangers Fear of being alone Fear of animal	
Insomnia	Difficulty falling asleep or staying asleep Difficulty with nightmares	
Intellectual impairment	Poor concentration Memory impairment	
Depressed mood	Decreased interest in activities Anhedonia Insomnia	
Somatic complaints: Muscular	Muscle aches or pains Bruxism	
Somatic complaints: Sensory	Tinnitus Blurred vision	
Cardiovascular symptoms	Tachycardia Palpitations Chest pain Sensation of feeling faint	
Respiratory symptoms	Chest pressure Choking sensation Shortness of breath	
Gastrointestinal symptoms	Dysphagia Nausea or vomiting Constipation Weight loss Abdominal fullness	
Genitourinary symptoms	Urinary frequency or urgency Dysmenorrhea Impotence	
Autonomic symptoms	Dry mouth Flushing Pallor Sweating	
Behaviour at interview	Fidgets Tremor Paces	
	Total score	

Phobias

Patients with phobias have the same symptoms as those with generalized anxiety disorder but symptoms are limited to specific situations. *Features:*
- *Avoidance* of the circumstances that provoke anxiety.
- *Anticipatory anxiety* when there is the prospect of encountering those circumstances.

Simple phobia: Inappropriate anxiety in the presence of ≥1 object/situation e.g. flying, enclosed spaces, spiders. Common in early life. Most adult phobias are a continuation of childhood phobias. *Lifetime prevalence:* 4% ♂; 13% ♀.

Management: Treatment is only needed if symptoms are frequent, intrusive or prevent necessary activities. Exposure therapy is effective. Obtain directly (via trained psychotherapist), by referral to psychiatry or through the private sector e.g. British Airways fear of flying course.

Social phobia: Intense and persistent fear of being scrutinized or negatively evaluated by others causing fear and avoidance of social situations (e.g. meeting people in authority, using a telephone, speaking to a group). Must be significantly disabling, not simple shyness. May be generalized (most social situations) or specific (certain activities only).

Management:
- *Drug therapy:* SSRIs—continue ≥ 12mo. *or* long-term if symptoms remain unresolved, co-morbid condition (depression, generalized anxiety disorder, panic attacks, history of relapse, or early onset.
- *Psychological therapies:* Cognitive behaviour therapy (cognitive restructuring) ± exposure. Obtain directly or via local psychiatric services depending on local arrangements.

Agoraphobia: Onset is usually aged 20–40y. and associated with an initial panic attack. Panic attacks, fear of fainting and/or loss of control are experienced in crowds, away from home or in situations from which escape is difficult. Avoidance → patients remaining within their home where they know symptoms will not occur. Other symptoms include depression, depersonalization and obsessional thoughts.

Management: Difficult to manage in general practice. Diagnosis is often delayed as patients will not come to the surgery and ongoing management is complicated by refusal to be referred to psychiatric services. Prognosis is best when there is good marital/social support. *Options:*
- *Behavioural therapy:* e.g. exposure, training in coping with panic attacks. Available by direct referral or via psychiatric services according to local arrangements. Home visits may be required, but should be resisted as part of therapy.
- *Drug treatment:* SSRIs (citalopram and paroxetine are licenced); MAOIs; TCAs (imipramine and clomipramine are commonly used). Relapse rate is high. Benzodiazepines can be used if frequent panic attacks particularly if initiating other treatment—but beware of dependence.

GP contract			
Indicators		**Points**	**Payment Schemes**
Records Indicator 9	For repeat medicines, an indication for the drug can be identified in the records (for drugs added to the repeat prescription with effect from 1 April 2004).	4 points	Minimum standard 80%

Advice for patients: Information and support for patients

Royal College of Psychiatrists: Patient information sheets
▨ www.rcpsych.ac.uk
Triumph Over Phobia (TOP) UK. Self-help materials and groups
☎ 01225 330 353 ▨ www.triumphoverphobia.com
No More Panic ▨ www.nomorepanic.co.uk

Acute panic attack

Features: Fear, terror and feeling of impending doom accompanied by some or all of the following:
- Palpitations
- Shortness of breath
- Choking sensation
- Dizziness
- Paraesthesiae
- Chest pain/discomfort
- Sweating
- Carpopedal spasm

Differential diagnosis
- Dysrhythmia
- Asthma
- Anaphylaxis
- Thyrotoxicosis
- Temporal lobe epilepsy
- Hypoglycaemia
- Phaeochromocytoma (very rare)

Action

Talking down: Explain the nature of the symptoms to the patient:
- Racing of the heart is due to adrenaline produced by the panic
- Paraesthesiae and feelings of dizziness are due to overbreathing due to panic
- Count breaths in and out gently slowing breathing rate.

Rebreathing techniques:
- Place a paper bag over the patient's mouth and ask him to breath in and out through the mouth.
- A connected but not switched on O_2 mask or nebulizer mask is an alternative in the surgery.
- This raises the partial pressure of CO_2 in the blood and symptoms due to low CO_2 (e.g. tetany, paraesthesiae, dizziness) resolve. This demonstrates the link between hyperventilation and the symptoms too.

Propranolol: 10–20mg stat may be helpful—**DON'T USE** for asthmatics or patients with heart failure or on verapamil.

Advice for patients: Self help

One way of tackling panic attacks is to look at the way you talk to yourself, especially during times of stress and pressure. Panic attacks often begin or escalate when you tell yourself scary things, like 'I feel light-headed … I'm about to faint!' or 'I'm trapped in this traffic jam and something terrible is gonna happen!' or 'If I go outside, I'll freak out.' These are called 'negative predictions' and they have a strong influence on the way your body feels. If you're mentally predicting a disaster, your body's alarm response goes off and the 'fight-flight response' kicks in.

To combat this, try to focus on calming, positive thoughts, like 'I'm learning to deal with panicky feelings and I know that people overcome panic all the time' or 'This will pass quickly, and I can help myself by concentrating on my breathing and imagining a relaxing place' or 'These feelings are uncomfortable, but they won't last forever.'

Remind yourself of these FACTS about panic attacks:
- A panic attack cannot cause heart failure or a heart attack.
- A panic attack cannot cause you to stop breathing.
- A panic attack cannot cause you to faint.
- A panic attack cannot cause you to 'go crazy.'
- A panic attack cannot cause you to lose control of yourself.

If it's too hard to think calming thoughts when you're having a panic attack, find ways to distract yourself. Some people do this by talking to other people when they feel the panic coming on. Others prefer to exercise or work on a detailed project or hobby. Changing scenery can sometimes be helpful, too, but it's important not to get into a pattern of avoiding necessary daily tasks. If you notice that you're regularly avoiding things like driving, going shopping, going to work, or taking public transport, it's probably time to get some professional help.

Slow, abdominal breathing (6 breaths per minute) has been shown to stop panic attacks. Learning slow abdominal breathing can be quite difficult and people who have panic attacks are almost always chest breathers. Practice abdominal breathing (moving upper part of tummy to breathe rather than chest wall) when relaxed at home. If you can learn to breathe slowly with your diaphragm, you will not panic!

Cut down on alcohol and caffeine—these can make panic attacks worse. Try relaxation techniques (such as yoga) and exercise regularly—both can help reduce the number of panic attacks people have.

Information and support for patients
Royal College of Psychiatrists: Patient information sheets
🖳 www.rcpsych.ac.uk
No More Panic 🖳 www.nomorepanic.co.uk

Panic disorder

Panic attacks are very common, but panic disorder is uncommon: lifetime prevalence 1% ♂; 3% ♀. NICE recommends a stepwise approach to management (Figure 3.6)

Step 1: Recognition and diagnosis

Symptoms: Patients experience intense feelings of apprehension or impending disaster. Anxiety builds up quickly and unexpectedly without a recognizable trigger and patients often present with any combination of:
- Shortness of breath and smothering sensations
- Choking
- Palpitations and accelerated heart rate
- Chest discomfort or pain
- Sweating
- Dizziness, unsteady feelings or faintness
- Nausea or abdominal pain
- Depersonalization/derealization
- Numbness or tingling sensations
- Flushes or chills
- Trembling or shaking
- Fear of dying
- Fear of doing something crazy or uncontrolled

Examination: Obvious distress; sweating; tachycardia; hyper-ventilation. ↑ BP is common and usually settles when the episode is over. Otherwise examination is normal.

Definitions:
- *Panic attack:* ≥4 symptoms listed above in 1 attack.
- *Panic disorder:* Chronic disorder; initial diagnosis depends on >4 attacks in 4wk. *or* 1 attack followed by a persistent fear of having another.

Differential diagnosis: Alcohol withdrawal; other psychiatric disorders (e.g. psychosis); hyperthyroidism; temporal lobe epilepsy; cardiac arrythmia; labyrinthitis; hypoglycaemia; hyperparathyroidism; phaeo-chromocytoma (very rare).

Associations: Depression (56% patients are depressed); generalized anxiety; agoraphobia; substance abuse; suicide (↑risk). Panic attacks may predict future panic disorder and depression—especially if the presenting feature is chest pain.

Acute management of panic attack: 📖 pp.82–3

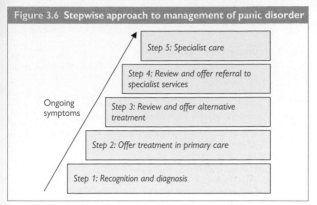

Figure 3.6 Stepwise approach to management of panic disorder

Ongoing symptoms

Step 5: Specialist care

Step 4: Review and offer referral to specialist services

Step 3: Review and offer alternative treatment

Step 2: Offer treatment in primary care

Step 1: Recognition and diagnosis

Step 2: Primary care management

⚠ Don't use benzodiazepines for treatment of patients with panic disorder—they are associated with less good outcome in the long term.

Consider treatment options

Psychological therapy: refer for CBT (📖 pp.100–1) ❶ often limited by availability in the community within a reasonable time frame.

Drug treatment: SSRIs e.g. escitalopram 5mg od and TCAs e.g. clomipramine 10–25mg nocte (unlicensed) are both effective (📖 p.60). SSRIs are usually used as first line treatment.

* Warn patients about possible transient ↑ in anxiety on starting treatment. GI side-effects are common. Tell patients they are unlikely to see improvements for 2wk. Minimize initial side-effects by starting at low dose and increasing slowly until there is a satisfactory response.
* Review <2wk. after starting treatment and at 4, 6, & 12 wk. If an SSRI is not suitable, or there is no improvement after 12 wk., offer imipramine or clomipramine (if appropriate) or another form of treatment.
* If effective, continue treatment for ≥6 mo. reviewing every 8–12wk. Minimize discontinuation symptoms by tapering dose over an extended time period

Self-help: Options are:

* Bibliotherapy based on CBT principles (📖 pp.100–1)
* Information about support groups
* Consider large group CBT where available
* Exercise—may benefit health generally
* Computerized CBT (📖 p.101)

Step 3: Review and offer alternative treatment: If treatment is complete and there has been no improvement, consider trying another type of intervention.

Step 4: Review and offer referral to specialist mental health services: If significant symptoms despite treatment with 2 different interventions (any combination of CBT, medication or bibliotherapy)

Essential reading

NICE Management of anxiety (panic disorder, with or without agoraphobia, and generalised anxiety disorder) in adults in primary, secondary and community care (2004) 🖥 www.nice.org.uk

GP contract			
Indicators		**Points**	**Payment Scheme**
Records Indicator 9	For repeat medicines, an indication for the drug can be identified in the records (for drugs added to the repeat prescription with effect from 1 April 2004).	4 points	Minimum standard 80%

GP Notes: Ways of improving outcome

Discuss treatment options: Shared decision-making between the individual and healthcare professionals improves concordance and clinical outcomes.

Provide information: Information in a form suitable to patients and/or carers about the nature, course and treatment of their anxiety disorder—including information on use and likely side effects of any medication—improves concordance and clinical outcomes.

Advice for patients: Information and support for patients

Anxiety Care Helpline ☎ 020 8478 3400 🖳 www.anxietycare.org.uk
No More Panic 🖳 www.nomorepanic.co.uk
Royal College of Psychiatrists: Patient information sheets
🖳 www.rcpsych.ac.uk

Obsessive-compulsive disorder (OCD)

Common mental illness characterized by recurrent obsessive thoughts and compulsive acts. Lifetime prevalence ~2% though minor obsessional symptoms are much more common. ♂:♀≈2:3. Onset tends to occur in adolescence (peak 12–14y.) or early adulthood (peak 20–22y.). There is often a family history and identical twin studies show ~90% concordance.

Theoretical basis: Cognitive behavioural theorists suggest obsessive thoughts generate anxiety which is partly relieved by certain actions; anxiety reduction reinforces the actions → development of compulsions.

Presentation: Onset may be acute or insidious and is associated with a precipitating event in 60%. Patients know obsessional thinking comes when what they are thinking or doing is irrational, making them embarrassed to tell anyone. As a result, patients may have had symptoms for years before seeking help. Relatives may highlight the problem rather than the patient. *Features:*

- *Obsessional thinking*—recurrent persistent thoughts (Have I turned the gas off?), impulses (e.g. to shout obscenities) and images (often of an obscene/violent nature) causing anxiety or distress.
- *Compulsive behaviour*—repetitive behaviours, rituals (e.g. handwashing, checking doors are locked) or mental acts done to prevent or ↓ anxiety.
- *Other features*—indecisiveness and inability to take action, anxiety, depression and depersonalization.

Diagnosis: For a diagnosis of OCD to be made:
- Obsessive thoughts/compulsive actions must be present on most days for ≥2wk.
- The patient must recognize that the thoughts come from within themselves (i.e. there are no passivity symptoms)
- Obsessive thoughts and compulsive rituals must have been unsuccessfully resisted in the past
- Thoughts and actions are unpleasant—if only due to repetition.

Differential diagnosis: Obsessive symptoms may occur as a result of a number of psychiatric conditions. It is important to distinguish OCD from such conditions. They are:
- Depression (~30% of severely depressed patients)
- Schizophrenia—suspect if thoughts or rituals are particularly bizarre
- Tourette's syndrome (📖 p.24)

Management: Refer for psychiatric assessment. Treatment involves a combination of patient education, SSRI, and/or CBT.

Prognosis:
- Most patients severely affected have a prolonged, steady course with symptoms decreasing slowly with time—2:3 improve within 1y. of presentation
- Symptoms worsen with stress
- 15% have a deteriorating course
- Bad prognostic indicators also include the presence of an obsessional personality and relative severity of symptoms.

Advice for patients: Patient experiences of OCD

'I'm afraid of catching something from other people, I fear that the germs that they carry may get on to me and I will become infected. I'm afraid I may also 'contaminate' my family by passing these germs on to them. I know it is silly but I feel so tense and anxious if I do touch anyone else or any surfaces—such as door handles that they have touched that I have to come home and wash my hands many times, then wash my clothes. That makes me feel a lot better until the next contact with others.'

'I fear that I will harm my partner, I know that I don't want to and I love her but thoughts often come into my head where I can picture myself harming her…with a knife or by strangling her. I am so upset when I have these thoughts that I have to bring into my mind other 'good thoughts' such as 'I know I love her very much' and I say these to myself many times to get rid of the bad thoughts. I usually feel a bit better after that, until the next time the awful thoughts come into my head. I have hidden away all sharp objects and knives so that there is no risk of me doing it and also seeing these objects brings the horrible thoughts to my mind.'

'My whole day is spent checking nothing will go wrong in the house … I can't get out because I'm never quite sure that I've turned off the gas, electric appliances, water and locked the windows…. I check to see if the gas fire is off, I do this 5 times and then can sometimes go upstairs, at other times it doesn't feel right and I go through the whole 'ritual' again. If I don't check I feel so worried I can't bear it…it's silly, but I keep thinking if something awful did happen I'd be to blame for being so careless.'

Self help strategy

- Carefully **recognize** your unwanted thoughts—**obsessions**—and the actions you take to put them right—**compulsions**.
- **Gradually** face some of the things you fear. Work out an anxiety ladder to help you do this (i.e. grade a list of unpleasant situations in terms of unpleasantness for you), begin with the easiest step.
- **Do not** carry out any compulsions to reduce or neutralize your anxiety when you are facing the feared situation.
- **Break** the obsession compulsion cycle.
- **Challenge** gloomy or critical thoughts you may have about yourself.

Information and support for patients

OCD Action ☎ 020 7226 4000 🖳 www.ocdaction.org.uk
Royal College of Psychiatrists: Patient information sheets
🖳 www.rcpsych.ac.uk

Further information:

NICE obsessive-compulsive disorder (2005) 🖳 www.nice.org.uk

Patient experience data and self-help strategy is reproduced with permission from the OCD information sheet available at 🖳 www.gp-training.net

Somatization and hysteria

Physical symptoms in response to emotional distress. Characterized by an excessive preoccupation with bodily sensations combined with a fear of physical illness. Common feature of depression, anxiety, schizophrenia, and substance use.

Somatization disorder: Chronic condition. History of numerous unsubstantiated physical complaints. Starts at <30y. and often persists many years. $\female$:$\male$≈10:1; lifetime prevalence 0.1–0.2% though mild symptoms are much commoner.

Clinical features:
- >2y. history of multiple symptoms with no adequate physical explanation.
- Persistent refusal to be reassured that there is no explanation for the symptoms.
- Impaired social/family functioning due to these symptoms and/or associated behaviour.

Management
- Reattribution: involves acknowledging and taking the symptoms seriously, offering any necessary examination and investigations, enquiring about psychosocial problems, and explaining the link between symptoms and stress.
- Treat co-morbid psychiatric problems (e.g. depression, anxiety, panic). ⚠ Beware of risks of drug interaction—self-medication with multiple OTC (or even prescription) drugs is common.
- Beware of side-effects of medication—patients do not tolerate prescribed drugs well and have a heightened awareness of side-effects.
- Refer to psychiatry if risk of suicide, marked functional impairment, impulsive or antisocial behaviour.

Munchausen syndrome (factitious disorder): Intentional production or feigning of physical or psychological symptoms to assume the sick role (± hospital admission). Can be difficult to detect. Differs from *malingering* as there is no external reward (e.g. financial) and from *somatization* in that it is deliberate. Associated with personality disorder.

Common presentations
- *Physical:* Dermatitis artefacta, pyrexia of unknown origin, bruising disorders, brittle DM, diarrhoea of unknown cause; neurological symptoms e.g. psudoparalysis or pseudofits (neurologica diabolica); abdominal pain (laparotomophilia migrans); chest pain (cardiopathia fantastica).
- *Psychological:* Feigned psychosis, fictitious overdose or bereavement.

Management
- Exclude any other basis for presenting pathology.
- Explain findings to the patient exploring possible causes.
- Assess psychological and social difficulties.
- Consider referral to psychiatry.

GP Notes: Heartsink patients

Characterized by
- Frequent presentation—the top 1% of attenders at GP surgeries generate 6% GP workload
- Highly complex and often multiple problems—some real, others not
- Exasperation generated between patient and doctor.

❶ It is a 2-way process. Some GPs report more heartsink patients than others. The problem relates to the GP's perception of patients as well as the patients themselves.

GP risk factors: Perception of high workload; low job satisfaction; lack of training in counselling or communication; lack of postgraduate skills.

Management
- Do a detailed review of notes ± chart of life
- Agree patient contacts e.g. limit to one partner, agree frequency of appointments etc.
- Agree an agenda within consultations e.g. problem list—only 1 problem/visit
- Employ reattribution techniques as for heartsink patients (see somatization disorder—📖 p.90).
- Avoid unnecessary investigation and referral
- Be aware of your own reaction to the patient
- Acknowledge even heartsink patients can be genuinely ill
- Consider psychiatric diagnoses—especially chronic anxiety, depression, somatization disorder. Screening questionnaires can be useful
- Consider referral for cognitive behavioural therapy.

91

Advice for patients: Information and support for patients and relatives

Self Injury and Related Issues (SIARI) 🖥 www.siari.co.uk

Munchausen syndrome by proxy: Caregiver—typically a mother with child—seeks repeated medical investigations and needless treatment for the person he/she is caring for. The child or person being cared for may actually be harmed by the carer to achieve these aims.

Common reported symptoms: Neurological, bleeding, rashes.

Management: Often difficult to detect and even harder to prove. A form of abuse that must be taken seriously and handled with care (📖 pp.46–9). Involve all relevant agencies early (e.g. social services, paediatrics).

Malingering: Intentional production or feigning of physical or psychological symptoms to assume the sick role for a known external purpose. Malingering is not considered mental illness or psychopathology, although it can occur in the context of other mental illnesses. *Forms:*
- *Pure malingering:* the individual falsifies all symptoms
- *Partial malingering:* the individual has symptoms but exaggerates the impact they have upon daily functioning
- *Simulation:* the individual acts out the symptoms of a specific disability
- *False imputation*—the individual has valid symptoms but is dishonest as to the source of the problems e.g. attributing neck pain to a road accident in order to obtain compensation.

Differential diagnosis
- True medical or psychiatric illness yet to be diagnosed
- Factitious disorder/Munchausen syndrome
- Somatization disorder.

Common motivating factors
- Avoidance of going to jail or release from jail
- Avoidance of work
- Avoidance of family responsibility
- Desire to obtain narcotics
- Desire to be awarded money in litigation
- Need for attention.

Management: Difficult. As doctors we tend to believe our patients.
- Exclude causes for the presenting symptoms through careful history/examination
- Avoid prescribing drugs for symptoms, and unnecessary referrals, as these might perpetuate symptoms
- Avoid certifying the patient as unfit to work or perform activities—if the patient is unhappy about this, suggest a second opinion
- Tactfully explain your findings and conclusions to the patient and explore the reasons for the behaviour.
- Provide support to find more appropriate ways to solve problems.

Chronic fatigue syndrome (CFS, ME)

A debilitating and distressing condition. *Prevalence*: 0.2–2.6%; ♀:♂ ≈ 3:2. *Cause*: Poorly understood—viral infections (≈10% after EBV), immunization, chemical toxins (e.g. organophosphates, chemotherapy drugs) are all implicated.

Clinical features: Unexplained fatigue of new/definite onset, not resulting from ongoing exertion, nor alleviated by rest, which results in ↓ activity, and ≥4 of:
- Impaired memory or concentration.
- Tender cervical/axillary lymph nodes.
- Postexertional malaise lasting >24 h.; typically delayed—usually starting 1–2d. after a period of ↑ physical/mental activity—and may last weeks.
- Headaches of new type pattern or severity.
- Multi-joint pain without swelling.
- Sore throat.
- Unrefreshing sleep.
- Muscle pain.

🚫 Additional symptoms must not have pre-dated fatigue

Other common symptoms /associations
- Postural dizziness
- Vertigo
- Altered temperature sensation
- Paraesthesiae
- Sensitivity to light or sound
- Palpitations
- IBS
- Food intolerance
- Fibromyalgia
- Feelings of dyspnoea
- Mood swings
- Panic attacks
- Depression (60% have no prior psychiatric diagnosis)

Intercurrent infection, immunization, drugs, caffeine, alcohol and stress may → setbacks.

Management
- Support and reassurance—explanation, information ± self-help groups
- Avoid factors which worsen symptoms e.g. caffeine, alcohol
- Graded exercise is helpful[C]
- Treat symptoms e.g. TCA (e.g. amitriptyline 10–50mg nocte) to help sleep, relieve headache or neuropathic pain; SSRI for depression
- Referral for specialist care e.g. CBT (↓ 2° distress and optimizes rehabilitation), specialist CFS clinic.

Prognosis: Variable. Children tend to recover though it may take years. 55% of adults presenting with tiredness have symptoms lasting >6 mo. Risk ↑ 3x if there is a history of anxiety or depression. Short duration of fatigue with no anxiety/depression improves prognosis. Only 6% of adults with CFS attending specialist clinics, return to pre-morbid functioning.

Further information
Royal Australian College of Physicians Chronic Fatigue Syndrome
🖳 www.mja.com.au/public/guides/cfs/cfs1.html
Kings College 🖳 www.kcl.ac.uk/cfs

Advice for patients: Information and support for patients

ME Association ☎ 0870 444 1836 🖳 www.meassociation.org.uk
Action for ME ☎ 0845 123 2380 🖳 www.afme.org.uk
Royal College of Psychiatrists: Patient information sheets
🖳 www.rcpsych.ac.uk

Eating disorders

⚠ Patients who are pregnant or have DM are particularly at risk of complications if they have co-morbid eating disorders. Refer early for specialist support and ensure everyone involved in care is aware of the eating disorder.

Anorexia nervosa: Prevalence 0.02–0.04%. ♀>>♂. Usually begins in adolescence. Peak prevalence at 16–17y. *Features:*
- Refusal to maintain body weight >85% of that expected (BMI <17.5 kg/m^2)
- Intense fear of gaining weight, though underweight
- Disturbed experience of body weight or shape or undue influence of shape on self-image
- Amenorrhoea in women for ≥3 mo. and ↓ sexual interest.

Patients tend to have a set daily calorific intake e.g. 600–1000 calories and may employ strategies e.g. bingeing and vomiting, purging or excessive exercise to try to lose weight. Depression and social withdrawal are common as are symptoms 2° to starvation (see above).

Management[N]
- Give ongoing support and information.
- Check electrolytes.
- Refer to a specialist eating disorders clinic (if available) or psychiatry. Treatment involves family therapy for adolescents, psychotherapy, and possible admission for refeeding.

Follow up: Patients with enduring anorexia nervosa not under 2° care follow up should be offered an annual physical and mental health check.

⚠ Many patients with anorexia nervosa have compromised cardiac function. Avoid prescribing drugs which adversely affect cardiac function (e.g. antipsychotics, TCAs, macrolide antibiotics, some antihistamines). If prescribing is essential then follow up with ECG monitoring

Binge eating disorder: A pattern of consumption of large amounts of food, even when a patient is not hungry. Common. Usually associated with obsessive feelings about food and body image, feelings of guilt/disgust about the amounts consumed and/or a feeling of lack of control.

Management
- Give ongoing support and information
- Provide an evidence-based self-help programme as a first step and/or antidepressant medication (SSRI is the drug group of choice).
- If unsuccessful refer for specialist help. CBT might be helpful.
- In all cases, provide concurrent advice and support to tackle any co-morbid obesity.

Target groups for screening include:

- Young women with low BMI compared with age norms
- Patients consulting with weight concerns who are not overweight
- Women with menstrual disturbances or amenorrhoea
- Patients with GI symptoms
- Patients with symptoms/signs of starvation—sensitivity to cold, delayed gastric emptying, constipation, ↓ BP, bradycardia, hypothermia.
- Patients with physical signs of repeated vomiting—pitted teeth ± dental caries, general weakness, cardiac arrythmias, renal damage, ↑ risk of UTI, epileptic fits, ↓K^+
- Children with poor growth
- Young people with type 1 DM and poor treatment adherence

Screen target populations with simple screening questions

- Do you worry excessively about your weight?
- Do you think you have an eating problem?

Advice for patients: Information and support for patient and parents

Eating Disorders Association (EDA) ☎ 0845 634 1414 (Adults) 0845 634 7650 (Youths) ▯ www.edauk.com

Essential reading

NICE Core interventions in the treatment and management of anorexia nervosa, bulimia nervosa and related eating disorders (2004) ▯ www.nice.org

Bulimia nervosa: Prevalence 1–2%. Mainly ♀ aged 16–40y. *Features:*
- Recurrent episodes of binge eating, far beyond normally accepted amounts of food.
- Inappropriate compensatory behaviour to prevent weight ↑ e.g. vomiting; use of laxatives, diuretics and/or appetite suppressants. Bulimics can be subdivided into those that purge and those that just use fasting and exercise to control their weight.
- Self-image unduly influenced by body shape (see Anorexia above).
- Normal menses and normal weight. If low BMI classified as anorexia.

Management
- Give ongoing support and information.
- Check electrolytes.
- First line treatment:
  - Evidence-based self-help programme e.g. Overcoming bulimia—CD-ROM available from Calipso ⊟ www.calipso.co.uk, telephone-based self-help programme run by the Eating Disorders Association—details below; cost ~£200 *and/or*
  - Antidepressant medication—fluoxetine 60mg od is the drug of choice
- If unsuccessful, refer to a specialist eating disorders clinic (if available) or psychiatry. CBT may help.

Advice for patients purging
- *Vomiting:* Advise patients to avoid brushing their teeth after vomiting, rinse with a non-acid mouthwash after vomiting, and ↓ acid oral environment (e.g. by limiting acid foods)
- *Laxatives:* Where laxative abuse is present, advise patients to gradually ↓ laxative intake. Laxative abuse does not significantly ↓ calorie absorption.

Essential reading
NICE Core interventions in the treatment and management of anorexia nervosa, bulimia nervosa and related eating disorders (2004) ⊟ www.nice.org

Advice for patients: Information and support for patient and parents

Eating Disorders Association (EDA) ☎ 0845 634 1414 (Adults) 0845 634 7650 (Youths) 🖥 www.edauk.com

Counselling and cognitive behaviour therapy

Counselling: 1:3 problems brought to the GP have a psychosocial component. To cater for these patients most PCOs (81%) have some provision for practice based counselling and 50% practices have counselling services. Counselling services may also be available via community psychiatric or clinical psychology services.

Table 3.3 Conditions suitable for referral to a counsellor

Conditions suitable for referral for counselling	Conditions unsuitable for referral
Anxiety	Psychotic illness
Depression—especially minor depression (📖 p.56)	Phobias
Relationship problems	Obsessive-compulsive disorder
Bereavement	Eating disorder
After traumatic events	Personality disorder
Substance abuse	

Problem-solving therapy: Another short-term therapy (typically 5–6 x 45 min. sessions) which involves drawing up a list of problems, and generating and agreeing solutions, broken down into steps, for patients to work on as homework between sessions (Figure 3.1, 📖 p.61). Shown to be as effective as antidepressants for moderate depression[R].

Cognitive behavioural therapy (CBT)

- *Behavioural therapies* aim to change behaviour. Usually the therapist uses a system of graded exposure (systematic desensitization) combined with teaching a method of anxiety reduction.
- *Cognitive therapy* focuses on peoples' thoughts and the reasoning behind their assumptions on the basis that incorrect assumptions → abnormal reactions which then reinforce these assumptions further (a vicious cycle).

Table 3.4 Recognized professional bodies in the UK

Counsellors
- The British Association for Counselling and Psychotherapy (BACP)
- The UK Register of Counsellors
- The Association of Counsellors and Psychotherapists in Primary Care

Psychologists
- The British Psychological Society (chartered and counselling psychologists)

Psychotherapists
- The UK Council for Psychotherapy
- The British Confederation of Psychotherapists

What is counselling? There are no universally agreed definitions of the term 'counselling' or 'counsellor' and the distinction between counselling and psychotherapy is often unclear. Usually the key element in counselling is reflective listening to encourage patients to think about and try to resolve their own difficulties. It does not involve giving advice. Most counsellors use brief (time-limited) therapy offering patients a mean of 7 sessions each usually lasting ~50 mins.

Who is a counsellor? There is no formal registration requirement in the UK for counsellors or psychotherapists. The GMC advises that GPs should only refer to practitioners who are members of a recognized disciplinary body and thus subject to ethical and disciplinary codes (Table 3.4).

Does counselling work? Many patients regard antidepressants as harmful or addictive and are increasingly reluctant to take them. They see counselling as an attractive alternative—a view supported by most GPs. Evidence shows counselling subjectively improves the condition the patient has been referred for and non-directive counselling is more effective than GP care in reducing anxiety and depression in the short-term but not the long-term. However, counselling doesn't ↓ drug costs and practices with counsellors make more referrals to 2° care psychiatric services[S]. More research is needed into cost-effectiveness.

Who should be referred? Counsellors see a wide range of patients (Table 3.3). $\sim^2/_e$ patients referred for counselling have significant levels of anxiety or depression.

What is CBT used for? CBT is of proven effectiveness in the treatment of mild depression, anxiety disorders, phobias, panic disorder, eating disorders and for the treatment of delusions and hallucinations in psychotic illness.

How can patients be referred for CBT? CBT is usually provided by highly trained psychotherapists and accessed via psychiatry services. Guided self-help programmes based on CBT are also effective for mild depression and can be delivered:
- Using books e.g. Gilbert *Overcoming depression* Constable and Robin (2000) ISBN: 1841191256
- By computer e.g. *Beating the Blues*[©] (further information available from 🖥 www.ultrasis.com), or
- Via the Internet e.g. 🖥 www.psychologyonline.co.uk

Further information
Bower *et al*. The clinical effectiveness of counselling in primary care (2003) **Psychol Med 33**: 203–15.

Alcohol misuse

Assessing drinking

Suspicious signs/symptoms: ↑ and uncontrolled BP; excess weight; recurrent injuries/accidents; non-specific GI complaints; back pain; poor sleep; tired all the time.

Ask: Assess amount, time of day, socially or alone, daily or in binges, blackouts, situations associated with heavy drinking. Consider using the CAGE questionnaire to assess dependence:
- Have you ever felt you should **C**ut down on your drinking?
- Have people **A**nnoyed you by criticizing your drinking?
- Have you ever felt bad or **G**uilty about your drinking?
- Have you ever had a drink first thing in the morning to steady your nerves or to get rid of a hang over (**E**ye opener)?

Risk factors
- Previous history
- Family history
- Poor social support
- Work absenteeism
- Emotional and/or family problems
- Financial and legal problems
- Drug problems
- Alcohol associated with work e.g. publican

Examination: Smell of alcohol, tremor, sweating, slurring of speech, BP (↑ BP); signs of liver damage.

Investigations: FBC (↑ MCV); LFTs (↑ GGT identifies ~25% of heavy drinkers in general practice; ↑ AST; ↑ bilirubin). Often incidental findings.

Health risk: Continuum—individual risk depends on other factors too (e.g. smoking, heart disease, pregnancy). Recommended safe levels of alcohol consumption are <21u/wk. for men and <14u./wk. for women. Alcohol-related health health problems—Table 3.6.

Table 3.5 Health risks associated with levels of alcohol consumption		
Health risk	**Men (units/wk.)**	**Women (units/wk.)**
Low	<21	<14
Intermediate	21–50	15–35
High	>50	>35

1 unit = 8g alcohol = 1/2 pint of beer (if strong beer can be as much as 1.75 units), small glass of wine/sherry, 1 measure of spirits (spirit measure in Scotland is 1.2 units).
1 bottle of 12% wine = 9 units.

Beneficial effects of alcohol: Moderate consumption (1–3 u./d.) ↓ risk of non-haemorrhagic stroke, angina pectoris, and MI.

Table 3.6 Alcohol-related problems

Death: ~40,000 deaths/y. in the UK are directly caused by alcohol.

Social

- Marriage breakdown
- Absence from work
- Loss of work
- Social isolation
- Poverty
- Loss of shelter/home

Mental health: Anxiety, depression and/or suicidal ideas; dementia and/or Korsakoffs ± Wernicke's encephalopathy

Physical

- ↑ BP
- CVA
- Sexual dysfunction
- Brain damage
- Neuropathy
- Myopathy
- Cardiomyopathy
- Infertility
- Gastritis
- Pancreatitis
- DM
- Obesity
- Fetal damage
- Haemopoietic toxicity
- Interactions with other drugs
- Fatty liver
- Hepatitis
- Cirrhosis
- Oesophageal varices ± haemorrhage
- Liver cancer
- Cancer of the mouth, larynx and oesophagus
- Breast cancer
- Nutritional deficiencies
- Back pain
- Poor sleep
- Tiredness
- Injuries due to alcohol-related activity (e.g. fights)

Advice for patients: Sources of advice and support

Drinkline (government-sponsored helpline) ☎ 0800 917 8282
Alcohol Concern 🖥 www.alcoholconcern.org.uk
Alcoholics Anonymous ☎ 0845 7697555
🖥 www.alcoholics-anonymous.org.uk

Alcohol management strategies: Figure 3.7.

Patients drinking within acceptable limits: reaffirm limits.

Non-dependent drinkers: Brief GP intervention results in ~24% reducing their drinking. Provide information about safe amounts of alcohol and harmful effects of exceeding these. If receptive to change, confirm weekly consumption using a drink diary, agree targets to ↓ consumption and negotiate follow-up.

Alcohol-dependent drinkers: Suffer withdrawal symptoms if they ↓ alcohol consumption (e.g. anxiety, fits, delirium tremens—see p.105, opposite).
- If wanting to stop drinking—refer to the community alcohol team; suggest self-help organizations e.g. Alcoholics Anonymous; involve family and friends in support.
- Detoxification in the community usually uses a reducing regimen of chlordiazepoxide over a 1 wk. period (20–30mg qds on days 1 and 2; 15mg qds on days 3 and 4; 10mg qds on day 5; 10mg bd on day 6; 10mg od on day 7 then stop).
- Community detoxification is contraindicated for patients with:
  - Confusion or hallucinations
  - History of previously complicated withdrawal (e.g. withdrawal seizures or delirium tremens)
  - Epilepsy or fits
  - Malnourishment
  - Severe vomiting or diarrhoea
  - ↑ risk of suicide
  - Poor co-operation
  - Failed detoxification at home
  - Uncontrollable withdrawal symptoms
  - Acute physical or psychiatric illness
  - Multiple substance misuse
  - Poor home environment.

If ambivalent/unwilling to change: provide information; reassess and re-inform on each subsequent meeting; support the family.

Vitamin B supplements: People with chronic alcohol dependence are frequently deficient in vitamins, especially thiamine—give oral thiamine indefinitely (if severe 200–300mg/d.; if mild 10–25mg/d.)[G]. During detoxification in the community—give thiamine 200mg od for 5–7d.

Relapse: Common. Warn patients and encourage them to re-attend. Be supportive and maintain contact (↓ frequency and severity of relapses[G]). Consider drugs to prevent relapse e.g. acamprosate, disulfiram (specialist initiation only).

Alcohol and driving: 📖 p.143

Essential reading

BMJ *Addiction and dependence—II: alcohol.* (1997)315, 358–360.
DTB *Managing the heavy drinker in primary care.* (2000) 38(8), 60–64.
SIGN *The management of harmful drinking and alcohol dependence in primary care.* (2003) 🖥 www.sign.ac.uk

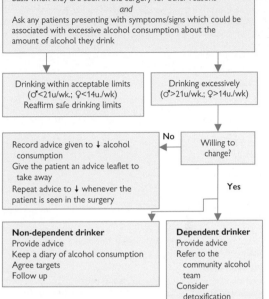

Figure 3.7 Alcohol management strategy

Assess the amount of alcohol patients are drinking on a regular basis when they are seen in the surgery for other reasons

and

Ask any patients presenting with symptoms/signs which could be associated with excessive alcohol consumption about the amount of alcohol they drink

Drinking within acceptable limits (♂<21u./wk.; ♀<14u./wk)
Reaffirm safe drinking limits

Drinking excessively (♂>21u./wk.; ♀>14u./wk)

Willing to change?

No

Record advice given to ↓ alcohol consumption
Give the patient an advice leaflet to take away
Repeat advice to ↓ whenever the patient is seen in the surgery

Yes

Non-dependent drinker
Provide advice
Keep a diary of alcohol consumption
Agree targets
Follow up

Dependent drinker
Provide advice
Refer to the community alcohol team
Consider detoxification

⚠ **Delirium tremens (DTs)**

Major withdrawal symptoms usually occur 2–3 d. after an alcoholic has stopped drinking. *Features:*
- *General:* Fever, tachycardia, ↑BP, ↑ respiratory rate
- *Psychiatric:* Vivid visual and tactile hallucinations, acute confusional state, apprehension
- *Neurological:* Tremor, fits, fluctuating level of consciousness

Action: DTs have 15% mortality and always warrant emergency hospital admission.

Drug misuse

1:10 adults report using illicit drugs in the last year. Of those presenting for treatment opioids are the main drugs of abuse (heroin: 54%; methadone: 13%) but the most frequently abused drugs are cannabis, amphetamine, ecstasy and cocaine. 3 factors appear important:

- availability of drugs;
- vulnerable personality; and
- social pressures—particularly from peers.

Detection: warning signs suggesting drug misuse include:

Use of services: Suspicious requests for drugs of abuse (e.g. no clear medical indication, prescription requests are too frequent).

Signs and symptoms
- Inappropriate behaviour
- Lack of self-care
- Unexplained nasal discharge
- Unusually constricted or dilated pupils
- Evidence of injecting (e.g. marked veins)
- Hepatitis or HIV infection.

Social factors: family disruption, criminal history.

Assessment: Assess on >1 occasion before deciding how to proceed. Exceptions are severe withdrawal symptoms and/or evidence of an established regime requiring continuation. Points to cover:

General information
- Check identification (ask to see an official document)
- Contact with other agencies (including last GP)—check accuracy of report
- Current residence
- Family—partner, children
- Employment
- Finances
- Current legal problems
- Criminal behaviour—past and present.

History of drug use: Current and past usage; knowledge of risks; unsafe sexual practices.

Medical and psychiatric history
- Complications of drug abuse e.g. HIV, hepatitis, accidents
- General medical and psychiatric history
- Overdoses—accidental or deliberate
- Alcohol abuse.

Investigations: Consider urine toxicology to confirm drug misuse; blood for FBC, LFTs, Hepatitis B, C, & HIV serology (with consent and counselling).

GMS contract

Specialized care of patients suffering from drug misuse may be
provided by practices as a National enhanced service—📖 pp.170–1

Advice for patients: Advice and support for drug misusers

'Talk to FRANK' (England and Wales) Government-run
information, advice and referral service. ☎ (24 hour) 0800 77 66 00
🖥 www.talktofrank.com
'Know the Score' (Scotland) ☎ 0800 587 5879
🖥 www.knowthescore.info
Drugscope Information about drug abuse and how to get treatment
🖥 www.drugscope.org.uk
Drugs-info Information about substance abuse for families of addicts
🖥 www.drugs-info.co.uk
ADFAM Support for families of addicts. ☎ 020 7928 8898
🖥 www.adfam.org.uk
Ecstasy 🖥 www.ecstasy.org
Benzodiazepines 🖥 www.benzo.org.uk
Solvent abuse ☎ 0808 800 2345 🖥 www.re-solv.org
National Treatment Agency for Substance Abuse 🖥 www.nhs.uk
Substance Misuse Management in General Practice (SMMGP)
🖥 www.smmgp.demon.co.uk/index.htm

Management of drug misuse. *Aims to:*
- ↓ risk of infectious diseases
- ↓ drug-related deaths
- ↓ criminal activity used to finance drug habits

The GP and PHCT have a vital role—identifying drug misusers; assessing their health and willingness to modify drug abusing behaviour; and, routine screening and prevention (e.g. cervical screening, contraception).

General measures. At each meeting consider:

Education
- Safer routes of drug administration
- Risks of overdose
- Condom use
- Driving and drug misuse (📖 p.143)

Hepatitis B immunization: for injecting drug misusers not already infected/immune and close contacts of those already infected.

Treatment of dependence
- Set realistic goals
- Responsibility contracts signed by GP, patient ± community pharmacist can be helpful.
- Review regularly
- Give contact numbers for community support organizations (📖 p.176)
- Seek advice and/or refer to a Community Substance Misuse Team as needed.

Specific drugs: Table 3.7

Solvent abuse
- Common amongst teenagers as solvents are easily obtained and cheap.
- Initial effects of inhalation are euphoria, incoordination, blurred vision and slurring of speech.
- Rarely the solvent may cause bronchoconstriction or arrhythmia and deaths, when they occur, are usually due to hypoxia, VF, or accidents whilst intoxicated.
- Symptoms to look for in the surgery are changes in behaviour (e.g. drop in school performance or attendance, irritability, mood swings) and local changes due to inhalation (e.g. cough, headaches, conjunctivitis).
- If detected, refer to the youth support agencies.

Essential reading
DoH: Drug misuse and dependence—guidelines on clinical management (1999) 🖥 www.dh.gov.uk

Table 3.7 **Withdrawal of common drugs**

Drug class	Drug withdrawal effects	Action
Opiates	*Symptoms:* Sweating Running eyes/nose Hot and cold turns ± gooseflesh GI problems—anorexia, nausea, vomiting, diarrhoea, abdominal pain Restlessness and tremor Insomnia Aches and pains Tachycardia ± hypertension Untreated heroin withdrawal reaches a peak 36–72h. after the last dose (methadone—4–6d.) Symptoms subside by 5d (methadone—10–12d.)	Refer to substance abuse team.
Benzodiazepines	*Symptoms include:* Rebound anxiety Tremor Tachycardia Tachypnoea Nausea and/or diarrhoea Abdominal and muscular cramps Rarely perceptual disturbances and seizures	Taper dosage over weeks. Seek specialist advice if the patient has any chronic debilitating condition or heart disease.
Stimulants (e.g. amphetamines, cocaine, ecstasy)	Some patients experience insomnia and depression. May require antidepressant drugs after withdrawal.	Can be stopped abruptly.
Hallucinogenic drugs (e.g. LSD)		Can be stopped abruptly.
Barbiturates	Sudden cessation may cause fits ± death.	Admit to hospital for supervised withdrawal.

Psychosis

The archetypal layman's 'madness'. Characterized by a loss of the link between reason and the outside world. Psychosis is not a diagnosis but a class of illnesses characterized by 3 key features:

- Hallucinations—📖 p.18
- Delusions—📖 p.18 *and*
- Thought disorder—📖 pp.18–19

If ≥1 of these features is present diagnosis is very limited:

- ***Affective psychoses***—psychotic depression, mania and hypomania (below)
- ***Delusional psychosis***—schizophrenia and paranoid psychoses (📖 pp.18–19, 114–17) *or*
- ***Organic psychoses***—the dementias (📖 pp.120–5), acute confusional states (📖 pp.118–19).

Mania and hypomania

Mania is characterized by a persistently high or euphoric mood out of keeping with circumstances. Other signs include:

- ↑ pressure of speech
- ↑ energy and activity
- ↑ appetite
- ↑ sexual desire
- ↑ pain threshold
- ↓ desire or need for sleep
- ↓ insight
- Grandiose delusions
- Hallucinations
- Spending sprees
- Disinhibition
- Self-important ideas
- Poor concentration—easily distracted
- Labile mood—elation → irritability/hostillity when thwarted
- Over-assertiveness

Hypomania is a less severe form of mania.

Differential diagnosis

- Hypoglycaemia
- Alcohol or drug abuse
- Prescribed drug side effects (e.g. steroids)
- Temporal lobe epilepsy
- Frontal lobe dysfunction (e.g. due to tumour or stroke)
- Thyrotoxicosis.

Acute management

Treatment in hospital is usually required for the 1st episode or acute relapses. If unwilling to accept voluntary admission, use compulsory admission under the Mental Health Act (📖 pp.134–7). Sedation whilst awaiting admission may be required—use chlorpromazine 50–100mg po or 50mg im (↓ dose for elderly patients and avoid if the patient is epileptic, has been drinking or taking barbiturates).

Advice for patients: Information and support for patients

Manic Depression Fellowship ☎ 020 8974 6550
▢ www.mdf.org.uk
Royal College of Psychiatrists: Patient information sheets
▢ www.rcpsych.ac.uk

Chronic management: Requires long-term follow-up:
- *Regular reviews:* Case registers help ensure regular reviews take place. Check a written care plan has been drawn up by the psychiatric service. Assess symptoms; compliance with medication; efficacy of treatment; medication side-effects; risks of suicide.
- *Educate* the patient and relatives/friends about early signs of relapse and action in case of relapse.
- *Reinforce compliance with treatment.*
- *Ensure adequate social support:* self-help groups, day centres, benefits
- *Monitor drugs for toxic side-effects.*
- *Advise patients to inform the DVLA:* driving should cease during the acute illness (all vehicles) and until stable with insight for three years (LGV/PCV drivers)—📖 pp.142–3.

Drug treatment: *BNF 4.2.3*
- Lithium is the drug of choice. It should only be initiated under specialist care.
- Check levels weekly until the dose is constant for 4wk., then monthly for 6 mo., then every 3–6mo. thereafter as long as the dose remains constant. Normal range is 0.6–1.0 mmol/l (though the elderly may be maintained at levels lower than this range)$^£$.
- If levels are slowly rising suspect nephrotoxicity.
- Check plasma creatinine, Ca^{2+} and TFTs every 6mo.$^£$
- Do not prescribe generically and avoid changing proprietary brands as bioavailability varies.
- *Toxic effects:* blurred vision, D&V, ↓K^+, drowsiness, ataxia, coarse tremor, dysarthria, hyperextension, fits, psychosis, coma and shock. Serum levels >1.5mmol/l can be fatal. If toxicity is suspected refer as an emergency for expert management.
- *Alternative drugs:* sodium valproate; carbamazepine.

Lithium monitoring: 📖 pp.166–7

Bipolar disorder or manic depression: Consists of episodes when the patient has mania (bipolar I) or hypomania (bipolar II) against a background of depression. Lifetime prevalence ≈1%. ♂:♀ ≈ 1:1. Peak incidence is in late teens and early 20's—90% develop the disorder before 30y.

Management: as for mania.

GP contract			
Indicator		**Points**	**Payment Scheme**
Mental Health Indicator 1	The practice can produce a register of people with schizophrenia, bipolar affective disorder or other psychosis	4 points	
Mental Health Indicator 2	The percentage of patients with schizophrenia, bipolar affective disorder or other psychosis	up to 23 points	Range 40–90%
Mental Health Indicator 4	The percentage of patients on lithium therapy with a record of serum creatinine and TSH in the preceding 15 mo.	up to 1 points	Range 40–90%
Mental Health Indicator 5	The percentage of patients on lithium therapy with a record of lithium levels in the therapeutic range within the previous 6 mo.	up to 2 points	Range 40 70%
Mental Health Indicator 6	The percentage of patients on the mental health register who have a comprehensive care plan documented in the records agreed between the individual their family and/or carers as appropriate	up to 6 points	Range 25–50%
Mental Health Indicator 7	The percentage of patients on the mental health register who do not attend the practice for their annual review, who are identified and followed up by the practice team ≤14d. after non-attendance	up to 3 points	Range 40–90%
Records Indicator 9	For repeat medicines, an indication for the drug can be identified in the records (for drugs added to the repeat prescription with effect from 1 April 2004).	4 points	Minimum standard 80%

GP Notes: Lithium treatment

A lithium treatment card available from pharmacies tells patients:
- How to take lithium preparations
- What to do if a dose is missed, *and*
- What side-effects to expect.

It also explains why regular blood tests are important and warns that some medicines and illnesses can change serum-lithium concentration

Cards may be obtained from NPA Services, 38–42 St. Peter's St, St. Albans, Herts AL1 3NP.

Schizophrenia

Frightening and disabling condition in which the sufferer is unable to distinguish his internal from the outside world. Lifetime prevalence ≈1%. Peak age of onset—♂ (15–25y.); ♀ (25–35y.).

First rank symptoms: Reliable markers in ~70% of patients. ≥1 symptom is suggestive of schizophrenia:
- Auditory hallucinations in the form of a commentary
- Hearing thoughts spoken aloud
- Hearing voices referring to the patient, made in the 3rd person
- Somatic hallucinations
- Thought broadcasting
- Thought withdrawal, insertion and interruption
- Delusional perception
- Feelings or actions experienced as made or influenced by external agents (passivity feelings).

Acute schizophrenia: Typically presents in a young people with +ve symptoms (delusions, hallucinations and/or thought disorder). The patient lacks insight so initial approach may come from a relative or friend.

Assessment: See the patient.
- Try to elicit any history of drug abuse—amphetamines can give a picture identical to schizophrenia.
- Ask about physical and psychological symptoms—in particular thoughts and perceptions.
- Assess the patient's behaviour and appearance. Look for evidence of self-care, loss of affect, poverty of thought and social withdrawal.
- Ask friends, neighbours or relatives present to tell you about of the patient's behaviour.

Differential diagnosis
- Illicit drugs
- Temporal lobe epilepsy
- Acute confusional state
- Dementia
- Affective disorders
- Personality disorder.

Management: Figure 3.8.

Follow up: Liaise with the community psychiatric services and reinforce the management plan agreed. Following acute episodes there is ↓ risk of relapse if antipsychotic medication continues 6–24 mo. Provide contacts for patient and relative support groups.

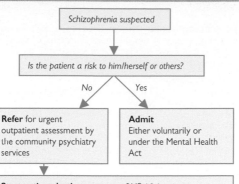

Figure 3.8 Acute management of schizophrenia

Schizophrenia suspected

Is the patient a risk to him/herself or others?

No — Yes

Refer for urgent outpatient assessment by the community psychiatry services

Admit Either voluntarily or under the Mental Health Act

Start antipsychotic treatment: *BNF 4.2.1*
Oral atypical antipsychotic drugs (e.g. amisulpride, olanzapine, risperidone) are 1st line treatment for newly diagnosed schizophrenia.

Stick to a single drug and start at the lower end of the dose range e.g. risperidone 1mg bd on day 1 and ↑ to 2mg bd on day 2.

Don't use loading doses.

❶ If necessary start antipsychotic treatment before psychiatric assessment—delay in treatment ↑ patient risks and → poorer prognosis

115

GP Notes: Schizophrenia and driving

⚠ Advise patients with schizophrenia who drive to inform the DVLA —driving should cease during the acute illness (all vehicles) and until stable with insight for 3y. (LGV/PCV drivers)—📖 pp.142–3

Chronic schizophrenia: Characterized by thought disorder and −ve symptoms (poverty of thought, apathy, inactivity, lack of volition, social withdrawal, and loss of affect). Aim to treat the disease, prevent relapse, and improve quality of life.

Long-term health problems
- ↑ death from suicide (1:10 schizophrenics), accidents, cardiovascular disease and respiratory disease.
- ↑ obesity due to side-effects of antipsychotic drugs, poor diet, sedentary lifestyle and lack of exercise.
- Substance abuse—¾ smoke; ↑ prevalence of alcohol and drug abuse.
- Rarely patients drink excessive amounts of water → hyponatraemia

Regular reviews[£]*:* Case registers ensure regular reviews take place.
- *Check there is a written care plan* from the psychiatric service.
- *Check mental health:* assess symptoms; compliance with medication; efficacy of treatment; medication side-effects; risks of suicide.
- *Check physical health:* watch for weight ↑, DM, and hyperprolactinaemia, especially on atypical antipsychotics. Check BP and lipids. ECG if palpitations—look for QT prolongation on atypical antipsychotics.
- *Promote lifestyle changes:* ↑ exercise; ↓ smoking; improve diet; encourage sensible drinking and avoidance of illicit drugs e.g. cannabis and amphetamines which exacerbate symptoms and ↑ risk of relapse.
- *Review social support:* areas where assistance may be needed include: finances, housing, employment, structured daily activity, transport, social network. Those who can help include: social services, community mental health team, housing officer, disablement resettlement officer.

Referral to Psychiatry: U=Urgent; S=Soon; R=Routine
- ↑ in risk to self or others—U
- Poor response to treatment—U/S/R
- Problems with adherence—consider depot administration—S/R
- Suspected co-morbid substance misuse—R
- Patient new to your practice—R
- Patient is on conventional antipsychotics (e.g. sulpiride, thioridazine) and suffering significant side-effects or persistent symptoms—refer for consideration of change of medication to atypical antipsychotic—R
- For family interventions to ↓ 'expressed emotion' (smothering, or hostility and criticism about the patient by the family)—effective in ↓ relapse—R
- For CBT—for persistent symptoms despite antipsychotics, and to ↑ insight—R

GP contract

Indicator		Points	Payment Scheme
Mental Health Indicator 1	The practice can produce a register of people with schizophrenia bipolar affective disorder or other psychosis.	4 points	
Mental Health Indicator 2	The percentage of patients with schizophrenia, bipolar affective disorder or other psychosis with a review recorded in the preceding 15 mo.	up to 23 points	Range 25–90%
Mental Health Indicator 6	The percentage of patients on the mental health register who have a comprehensive care plan documented in the records agreed between the individual their family and/or carers as appropriate	up to 6 points	Range 25–50%
Mental Health Indicator 7	The percentage of patients on the mental health register who do not attend the practice for their annual review, who are identified and followed up by the practice team ≤14d. after non-attendance	up to 3 points	Range 40–90%
Medicines Management Indicator 7	Where the practice has responsibility for administering regular injectable neuroleptic medication, there is a system to identify and follow up patients who do not attend	4 points	
Records Indicator 9	For repeat medicines, an indication for the drug can be identified in the records (for drugs added to the repeat prescription with effect from 1 April 2004).	4 points	Minimum standard 80%
Education Indicator 7	The practice has undertaken a minimum of 12 significant event reviews in the past 3 years which could include: A suicide A section under the Mental Health Act	4 points	For 12 audits

117

Advice for patients: Information and support for patients and relatives

National Association for Mental Health (MIND) ☎ 020 8519 2122
🖳 www.mind.org.uk
Rethink (National Schizophrenia Fellowship) ☎ 020 8974 6814
🖳 www.nsf.org.uk

Acute confusional states (delirium)

Common condition seen in general practice—particularly amongst elderly patients. May occur de novo or be superimposed upon chronic confusion of dementia (📖 pp.120–5) resulting in sudden worsening of cognition.

Presentation

- Global cognitive deficit with onset over hours/days
- Fluctuating conscious level—typically worse at night/late afternoon
- Impaired memory—on recovery amnesia of the events is usual
- Disorientation in time and place
- Odd behaviour—may be underactive, drowsy and/or withdrawn *or* hyperactive and agitated
- Disordered thinking—often slow and muddled ± delusions (e.g. accuse relatives of taking things)
- Disturbed perceptions—hallucinations (particularly visual) are common
- Mood swings.

Examination: Can be difficult. If possible do a thorough general physical examination to exclude treatable causes.

Possible causes: Table 3.8

Differential diagnosis

- Deafness: may appear confused
- Dementia: longer history and lack of fluctuations in conscious level—in practice may be difficult to distinguish especially if you come across a patient who is alone and can give no history
- Primary mental illness e.g. schizophrenia (📖 pp.114–17); anxiety state (📖 pp.74–9)

Management: Is aimed at treating all remediable causes.

Admit if:

- The patient lives alone
- The patient will be left unsupervised for any duration of time
- If carers (or residential home) are unprepared/unable to continue looking after the patient *and/or*
- If history and examination have indicated a cause requiring acute hospital treatment, admit as an emergency.

Possible investigations to consider in the community

- Urine: dipstick for glucose, ketones, blood, protein, nitrates and white cells, send for M,C&S
- BM to exclude hypoglycaemia
- Blood: FBC, ESR, U&E, LFTs, TFTs
- ECG
- CXR

Management at home
- Acute confusion is frightening for carers—reassure and support them.
- Treat the cause e.g. antibiotics for UTI or chest infection
- Try to avoid sedation as this can make confusion worse. Where unavoidable use haloperidol 1–2mg prn or lorazepam 0.5–1mg prn.
- Involve district nursing services e.g. to provide incontinence aids, cot sides, moral support.
- If the cause does not become clear despite investigation or the patient fails to improve with treatment admit for further investigation and assessment.

Table 3.8 Causes of acute confusional state

Infection	Particularly UTI, pneumonia; rarely encephalitis, meningitis
Drugs	Opiates, sedatives, L-dopa, anticonvulsants, recreational drugs
Metabolic	Hypoglycaemia, uraemia, liver failure, hypercalcaemia, other electrolyte imbalance (rarer)
Alcohol or drug withdrawal	
Hypoxia	e.g. severe pneumonia, exacerbation of COPD, cardiac failure
Cardiovascular	MI, stroke, TIA
Intracranial	Space occupying lesion, raised intracranial pressure, head injury (especially subdural haematoma)
Thyroid disease	Hyper- or hypothyroidism
Carcinomatosis	
Epilepsy	Temporal lobe epilepsy, post-ictal state
Nutritional deficiency	B_{12}, thiamine or nicotinic acid deficiency

Dementia

Generalized impairment of intellect, memory, and personality, with no impairment of consciousness. Prevalence ↑ with age (rare <60y.; 5% >65y.; 20% >80y.). *Common causes:* Alzheimer's disease (60%); vascular (multi-infarct) dementia; dementia with Lewy bodies.

Presentation

History: Patients may be aware of 'being a bit forgetful' but usually relatives complain about their behaviour. Early symptoms are loss of short-term memory and inability to perform normally simple tasks. Alternatively patients present later with failure to cope at home or self-neglect. To diagnose dementia there must be a clear history of progressive impairment of memory and cognition ± personality change.

Examination: Check general appearance—look for evidence of self-neglect, malnutrition, abuse; screen for cognitive deficit e.g. with the 6 Cognitive Impairment Test (🕮 p.6).

Investigation: Aimed at detecting treatable causes: check FBC, ESR, U&E, LFTs, Ca^{2+}, TFTs, glucose, B_{12}, red cell folate, VDRL (syphilis), HIV (if at risk), CXR, MSU.

Differential diagnosis
- Acute confusion: 🕮 pp.118–19
- Depression: 🕮 pp.56–65
- Communication problems: deafness, dysphasia or language difficulty.

Management
- *Refer:* All patients to a psychogeriatrician for confirmation of diagnosis, exclusion of treatable causes and ongoing specialist support and assessment. Refer to a social worker and/or CPN for community support.
- *Assess* level of support in the home, housing and ability to cope (both patient and carers). Refer for support as necessary.
- *Support carers* Listen to the carer, no-one knows more about their own situation than they do. Be aware of the full range of resources—advise re benefits, self-help groups, respite care. Warn that dementia is progressive and prepare carers for a time when the patient does not recognize them. ❶ Don't overlook the elderly isolated carer who makes few demands.
- *Treat concurrent problems* (e.g. UTI, chest infection, anaemia, depression)—they make dementia worse.
- *Management of memory loss:* Notebook to record 'tasks must do'; medication dispensers.
- *Management of agitation:*
  - Maintain a constant environment if possible
  - Arrange for door catches to prevent wandering
  - Take up loose carpets to prevent falls
  - Consider fire and electrical safety
  - Avoid sedatives wherever possible as may worsen confusion—if needed use very low dose, review regularly and consider newer atypical drugs e.g. risperidone.

GP contract			
Indicator		**Points**	**Payment Scheme**
Dementia 1	The practice can produce a register of patients diagnosed with dementia	5 points	
Dementia 2	The percentage of patients diagnosed with dementia whose care has been reviewed in the preceding 15mo. This should include an assessment of support needs of the patient and their carer and a review of co-ordination arrangements with secondary care.	up to 15 points	25–60%
Medicines Management Indicator 7	Where the practice has responsibility for administering regular injectable neuroleptic medication, there is a system to identify and follow up patients who do not attend	4 points	
Records Indicator 9	For repeat medicines, an indication for the drug can be identified in the records (for drugs added to the repeat prescription with effect from 1 April 2004).	4 points	Minimum standard 80%
Education Indicator 7	The practice has undertaken a minimum of 12 significant event reviews in the past 3 years which could include: A section under the Mental Health Act	4 points	For 12 audits

---

Advice for patients: Information and support for patients and carers

Alzheimer's Society ☎ 0845 300 0336 🖳 www.alzheimers.org.uk
Dementia Care Trust ☎ 0870 443 5325 🖳 www.dct.org.uk
DIPEx patient experience database 🖳 www.dipex.org
Benefits enquiry line ☎ 0800 882 200
Carers UK ☎ 0808 808 7777 🖳 www.carersonline.org.uk

Advice for patients: Carers' experiences of dementia

About dementia

- 'Dementia is like a continual bereavement, because unlike a proper bereavement where you have the great grief when you lose the person because they die … you're losing a bit of that person all the time and you're watching it happen. So day after day you're grieving for the bit, perhaps the next bit that's going, or the bit that suddenly comes to you that day.'

About the first signs of dementia

- 'The first insights that you have …a series of unrelated and apparently insignificant things that happen. It's only now that one can look back and make sense of them, so let me give you one or two examples … I remember saying to my wife 'Would you lock the car up and I'll go and get a parking ticket and then we'll go off.' We went off and came back an hour later and all the doors of the car had been left open. At the time we kind of laughed about it, no harm was done.'
- 'It had become evident… she was in some difficulty living on her own. She was falling out with people that she'd been friendly with a long time…for example putting her name down for an outing. She would say she didn't want to go so her name wouldn't be put on the list and then she would turn up for the bus with everybody else and be very upset that she wasn't allowed to get on it because she hadn't put her name down and there was no room. And she would say that she had put her name down and that somebody had crossed it off.'

About the carer's role

- 'I think another turning point was a realisation that…the carer is the expert. You know far more about the person you're caring for than all the doctors and the workers put together…. It's as though they all have bits of our jigsaw, but they don't have the picture on the box and the carer has the picture on the box and knows what it needs to look like.'
- 'You have to sort of look for things that will give you…pleasure on a, on a day-to-day basis. It may be just a walk in the park…small every-day things that just give you pleasure, both of you pleasure'
- 'You have to change your plans, your ideas, your timetable almost from minute to minute and I think that flexibility's quite important.'

About other people

- 'I think you've got to try to understand that perhaps the carer and other professionals are the only ones who can understand what the carer is actually experiencing. And we as carers should not expect that friends, relatives and other people will understand the situation that we are actually in.'

All quotes on this page are reproduced with permission of DIPEx ▥ www.dipex.org

About the carer's feelings

- 'I feel it's like a death without a funeral. But I would say to anyone who feels like this, "Don't ... dwell on the present when you feel depressed, don't dwell on the future, think of all the good times you've had, the places you've been, the things you've seen and shared" '.
- 'Admit to yourself how you feel... I have gone through all the negative emotions that a human being is able to go through. Anger, terrible, terrible anger at the whole situation...towards him personally and then the guilt, because it's not his fault. He didn't choose to be like this. In fact he'd be appalled if he could see himself.'

About the carer's health and well-being

- 'There are certainly times when you wonder if you're coping OK...it's very easy to run yourself into the ground, keep going at all costs and that cost might well be your own health.....you've got to take care of yourself otherwise you're not going to be in a position to carry on caring.'

About practical ways you can help yourself

- 'In hindsight I think that the carer should seek all the support that they possibly can from whoever is available ....whoever it is.'
- 'I think it would have helped if I could have joined, if I'd belonged to the local Carers' Association, but again I didn't know how to find it.'
- 'I started reading about dementia and understanding some of the problems then I could face ...I could face the situation a lot easier.'
- 'I think the big, the important thing I'd say to carers is "Tell people".I was amazed once I went round and started saying to people that I'd got a mother with dementia, how many other people were in this situation...there's an awful lot of people with knowledge and help. But unless you mention it, you don't find them.'
- 'The turning point for me was when I realized that I had to take the initiative and say "Look however bizarre it seems this is what pleases him. You know, at autumn time, he likes to go around on the grass, picking up interesting coloured autumn leaves"... And that to him was a meaningful—don't ask me why—a meaningful activity, far more meaningful than the bingo or whatever.'
- 'While the person concerned is still capable of doing things, get the Power of Attorney, try and get some opinions of what they want and try and get your finances sorted out.'
- 'I do think there should be a checklist somewhere of all these things that you are eligible for...if you're somebody who's very retiring and very shy and not one who's willing to get on the phone and find out you just sink...people who don't like to make a fuss, don't like to make waves, don't have much confidence, spend all their days looking after their partner or whatever and fall through the net.'

Alzheimer's disease: Most common form of dementia. Each GP has ~16 patients with Alzheimer's disease at any time. *Cause:* unknown—defective genes found on chromosomes 14, 19, and 21.

Risk factors: FH, Down's syndrome (onset at ~30y.), late onset depression, hypothyroidism, history of head injury.

Presentation: Presents with steady ↓ in memory and cognition. *Onset:* any age—normally >40y. ♀:♂ ≈ 0.7.

Management: Specific treatment with anticholinesterase inhibitors (e.g. donepezil, rivastimine) is now available. There is some evidence these drugs ↓ rate of decline. They are *only* prescribed for patients presenting with mild or moderate dementia and only under specialist supervision—refer.

Prognosis: Mean survival ~7y. from outset.

Lewy body dementia: Fluctuating but persistent cognitive impairment, parkinsonism and hallucinations. No specific treatment. Avoid antipsychotics as they can be fatal. Use benzodiazepines if tranquilization is necessary.

Pick dementia: Dementia characterized by personality change associated with frontal lobe signs such as gross tactlessness. Lack of restraint may lead to stealing, practical jokes and unusual sexual adventures. Treatment is supportive.

Vascular (multi-infarct) dementia: Multiple lacunar infarcts or larger strokes cause generalized intellectual impairment. Tends to occur in a stepwise progression with each subsequent infarct. The final picture is one of dementia, pseudobulbar palsy and shuffling gait with small steps. Secondary prevention of TIA/stroke ↓ the likelihood of further infacts and dementia progression.

GP Notes: ⚠ Beware of elder abuse

Elder abuse is defined as: 'A single or repeated act or lack of appropriate action, occurring within any relationship where there is an expectation of trust, which causes harm or distress to an older person'.

Older people may report the abuse but they often don't. It may take several forms which can co-exist:
- *Physical* e.g. cuts, bruises, unexplained fractures, dehydration/malnourishment with no medical explanation, burns
- *Psychological* e.g. unusual behaviour, unexplained fear, appears helpless or withdrawn
- *Financial* e.g. removal of funds by carers, new will in favour of carer
- *Sexual* e.g. unexplained bruising, vaginal or anal bleeding, genital infections
- *Neglect* e.g. malnourished, dehydrated, poor personal hygiene, late requests for medical attention

Prevalence (in own home): physical abuse—2%; verbal abuse—5%; financial abuse—2%.

Signs
- Inconsistent story from patient and carer
- Inconsistencies on examination
- Fear in the presence of the carer
- Frequent attendance at A & E
- Frequent requests for GP visits
- Carer avoiding the GP

Management
- Talk through the situation with the patient, carer, and other services involved in the elderly person's care.
- Assess the level of risk.
- Consider admission to a place of safety—contact social services and/or police as necessary.
- Seek advice from Action on Elder Abuse (☎ 0808 808 8141 🖫 www.elderabuse.org.uk).

125

Personality (behavioural) disorder

Patients may prefer the term 'personality difficulties'.

🄟 Personality changes rapidly through adolescence, and personality disorder should not be diagnosed aged <16–17 y.

Definition: Personality is defined as the enduring qualities of an individual shown in his or her ways of behaving in a wide variety of circumstances. Personality disorders are deeply ingrained patterns of behaviour which do not conform to the norms of society. *Features:*
- Pervasive and maladaptive patterns of behaviour, thinking, and control of emotions.
- These patterns of behaviour, thinking and control of emotions must be enduring and not limited to episodes of mental illness.
- There must be significant distress/disturbance in social function as a result of these patterns of behaviour

Diagnosis: Difficult. There is often significant overlap between symptoms of neurotic and/or psychotic illness and features of personality disorders. The problem is one of differentiating personality and illness. The key lies in the duration of the unusual behaviour—if the behaviour has always been abnormal or maladaptive then it is likely the patient has a personality disorder. If the patient has always behaved in a normal fashion and begins to behave abnormally—illness is likely.

🄟 A diagnosis of a personality disorder has huge implications for everyday life. Always refer for expert confirmation if personality disorder is suspected.

Classification: Table 3.9, 📖 pp.128–9

Management: A personality disorder is likely to remain fixed whatever treatment is tried. Management is largely practical, directed towards ameliorating the untoward effects of the disorder on the patient's life—rather than trying to change the patient's personality.
- Be clear about professional boundaries and avoid conflict.
- Involve family or friends in the care plan if appropriate
- Consider referral to psychiatry:
  - For diagnostic clarification
  - If there is a risk of harm to self or others
  - For treatment of co-morbid mental illness
  - For specialist treatment of personality disorder.
- SSRIs can help impulsive behaviour
- Low dose atypical antipsychotics may help paranoid ideas
- Mood stabilizers e.g. lithium may help emotional instability

⚠ Risk of overdose is ↑ amongst patients with personality disorder.

Advice for patients: Information and support for patients and relatives

Borderline UK 🖳 www.borderlineuk.co.uk
Borderline Personality Disorder (BPD) Central
🖳 www.bpdcentral.com

Table 3.9 ICD-10 categories of personality disorder

Category	Features
Paranoid	≥3 of: • Excessive sensitiveness to setbacks • Tendency to bear grudges persistently • Suspiciousness and tendency to misconstrue actions of others as hostile • Sense of personal rights out of keeping with the situation • Unjustified suspicions about infidelity of partner • Excessive self-importance • Unsubstantiated conspiratorial explanation of events.
Schizoid	≥3 of: • Few activities provide pleasure • Emotional coldness, detachment or flattened mood • Limited capacity to express good or bad feelings towards others • Apparent indifference to praise or criticism • Little interest in having sexual experiences with another person • Preference for solitary activities • Preoccupation with fantasy and introspection • Lack of close friends of desire for such relationships • Insensitivity to prevailing social norms and conventions.
Dissocial (antisocial)	Associated with criminal activity and antisocial behaviour. ≥3 of: • Lack of concern for the feelings of others • Irresponsibility and disregard for social norms, rules and obligations • Incapacity to maintain enduring relationships, though having no difficulty in establishing them • Easily frustrated and a low threshold for aggression/violence • Incapacity to experience guilt and to profit from experience, particularly punishment • Prone to blame others, or to offer plausible rationalizations, for antisocial behaviour • Persistent irritability may be an associated feature 🛈 Conduct disorder during childhood and adolescence further supports the diagnosis.
Emotionally unstable	
Impulsive type	• Emotional instability • Lack of self control • Characterized by violent/threatening outbursts particularly in response to criticism
Borderline type	• Emotional instability resulting in emotional crises • Unstable relationships • Self-image, aims and preferences are often unclear/disturbed • Chronic feelings of emptiness • Prone to suicidal threats/self-harm

Table 3.9 (Contd)

Category	Features
Histrionic	≥3 of: • Self-dramatization, exaggerated expression of emotions • Suggestible and easily influenced by others/circumstances • Shallow and labile mood • Continually seeks excitement, appreciation by others, and to be the centre of attention • Inappropriate seductiveness • Over-concern with physical attractiveness *Associated features include:* egocentricity, self-indulgence, longing for appreciation, easily hurt feelings, manipulative behaviour to achieve own needs.
Anakastic (obsessive-compulsive)	≥3 of: • Feelings of excessive doubt and caution • Preoccupation with details, rules, lists, order, organization or schedule • Perfectionism that interferes with task completion • Excessive conscientiousness to the exclusion of pleasure • Excessive adherence to social conventions • Rigidity and stubbornness • Unreasonable insistence that others do things exactly as the patient wants or unwillingness to allow others to do things • Intrusion of insistent and unwelcome thoughts or impulses.
Anxious (avoidant)	≥3 of: • Persistent feelings of tension and apprehension • Patient belief s/he is socially inept, unappealing or inferior • Preoccupation with being criticized or rejected • Unwillingness to become involved with people unless certain of being liked • Restrictions in lifestyle because of need to have physical security • Avoidance of activities involving significant interpersonal contact for fear of criticism, disapproval or rejection
Dependent	≥3 of: • Encouraging/allowing others to make important life decisions • Undue compliance and subordination to the wishes and needs of others • Unwillingness to make reasonable demands on others • Feeling uncomfortable, incompetent or helpless when alone • Preoccupation with fears of being abandoned • Limited capacity to make everyday decisions without advice/reassurance from others
Other specific	Includes *narcissistic personality disorder*: • Grandiose sense of self importance/uniqueness • Preoccupation with fantasies of unlimited success, power, brilliance, etc. • Lack of warmth and empathy • Often respond with rage provoked by criticism • Often exhibit boredom and emptiness.

129

ICD-10 classification of personality disorder reproduced with permission of the World Health Organization: ▣ www.who.int

Care for informal carers

In the UK there are 6 million informal carers who are vitally important to the wellbeing of disabled people in the community. Most are relatives or friends of the person being cared for. Many are elderly with health problems themselves. There is good evidence their health suffers as a result of caring—52% report treatment for a stress-related illness since becoming a carer and 51% report being physically injured as a result of caring.

GPs and their primary care teams are often the 1st point of access for any help needed and 88% of carers have seen their GP in the past 12 mo. Carers see the GP as the professional most able to improve their lives but few GPs have had any training about their problems and 71% carers believe their GPs are unaware of their needs.

Physical help: Record whether a patient is a carer in their notes.
- *Practical advice on nursing skills:* ask DNs to review problems.
- *Advice on management:* specialist nurses (e.g. CPNs etc.) provide special expertise.
- *Additional help:* social services can provide home care. Voluntary organizations provide sitting services e.g. Crossroads schemes. Every carer has a right to ask for a full assessment of their needs by the social services.
- *Home modification:* local authorities can arrange modifications. DNs have access to equipment needed for nursing. The Red Cross loans commodes, wheelchairs etc.
- *Respite:* hospitals, charity organizations and local authorities provide day care (to give regular breaks each week) and respite care (for a week or more at a time).

Emotional support
- *Self-help carers groups:* opportunity to share experiences with people in similar situations.
- *Always ask the carer how they are when visiting:* even if they are not your patient themselves.
- *If the patient and/or carer have a religion, the clergy will often provide ongoing support.*
- *Maintain good lines of communication.* Treat the carer as a team member. Make sure you inform both carer and patient fully. Make appointments for review. Don't be short with a carer, patronizing or impossible to contact.

Financial support: Many patients who have carers are entitled to Attendance Allowance or Disability Living Allowance (📖 p.156). If the patient is not expected to live >6mo. they are entitled to claim under Special Rules. This benefit is *not* means tested. Other benefits:
- *Low income:* 📖 pp.152–4
- *Given up work to look after the patient:* may be eligible for carer's allowance—📖 p.157.
- *Substantial modification to home:* council tax may be payable at lower rate (consult local council).

GP contract		
Indicator		**Points**
Management Indicator 9	The practice has a protocol for the identification of carers and a mechanism for the referral of carers for social services assessment	3 points

---

Advice for patients: Support organizations for carers

Carers UK ⌨ www.carersonline.org.uk ☎ 020 7490 8818
Princess Royal Trust for Carers ⌨ www.carers.org
☎ 020 7480 7788
Support organizations for the patient's condition
(e.g. Alzheimer's Society—📖 pp.176–9)
Department of Work and Pensions ⌨ www.dwp.gov.uk
☎ *Benefits Enquiry Line*—0800 882200; 0800 243355 (minicom facility); 0800 441144 (for help with form completion)
Citizens Advice Bureau ⌨ www.adviceguide.org.uk
Age Concern: ☎ 0800 00 99 66 ⌨ www.ageconcern.org.uk
Help the Aged: ☎ 0800 800 65 65 ⌨ www.helptheaged.org.uk
Counsel and Care ☎ 0845 300 7585
⌨ www.counselandcare.org.uk

Chapter 4

Legal aspects of mental health care in the community

Compulsory admission and treatment of patients with mental illness

Most requiring inpatient care for mental disorder agree to hospital admission and become 'informal' patients. A minority (~5%) require compulsory admission and detention under the Mental Health Act of 1983[1] and are termed 'Sectioned'—in reference to the Section of the Mental Health Act under which they are detained (Figure 4.1).

Procedure for 'sectioning' a patient

Applications can be made for
- Admission for assessment under Section 2 (📖 p.137)
- Admission for treatment under Section 3 (📖 p.137)
- Emergency admission under Section 4 (📖 p.137)
- Guardianship under Section 7 (📖 p.137).

Applications can be made by
- An approved social worker (ASW)
- The nearest relative of the person concerned. Nearest relative is defined in the Act as the 1st surviving person out of:
  - spouse (or co-habitee for >6mo.)
  - oldest child (if >18y.)
  - parent
  - oldest sibling (if >18y.)
  - grandparent
  - grandchild (>18y.)
  - uncle or aunt (>18y.)
  - nephew or niece (>18y.)
  - non-relative living with patient for ≥5y.

The applicant (ASW or nearest relative) must have seen the patient <2wk. (<24h. in the case of Section 4) before the date of the application.

🔔 The ASW should be chosen rather than the nearest relative wherever possible, to avoid affecting family relationships.

Applications must be based on
- 2 medical recommendations (except Section 4 which only needs 1). Doctors may examine the patient together or separately, but there must be <6d. between examinations. Recommendations must be signed on or before the date of application.
- Where 2 medical recommendations are required, the doctors should not be from the same hospital or practice *and* one of the doctors must be 'approved' under the Mental Health Act.
- One doctor, if practicable, must have prior knowledge of the patient (ideally a GP—but GPs are not obliged to attend outside the practice area). If neither doctor has prior knowledge of the patient, the applicant must state on the application why this was so.
- Medical recommendation(s) and application must concur on at least one form of mental disorder.

---

1 Applies in England and Wales only. In Northern Ireland similar provisions apply under the Mental Health (Northern Ireland) Order 1986. Scotland—see 📖 p.136

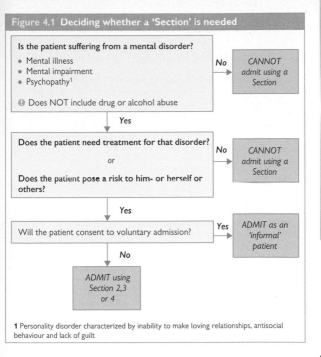

Figure 4.1 Deciding whether a 'Section' is needed

Is the patient suffering from a mental disorder?
- Mental illness
- Mental impairment
- Psychopathy[1]

ⓘ Does NOT include drug or alcohol abuse

→ **No** → *CANNOT admit using a Section*

↓ **Yes**

Does the patient need treatment for that disorder?

or

Does the patient pose a risk to him- or herself or others?

→ **No** → *CANNOT admit using a Section*

↓ **Yes**

Will the patient consent to voluntary admission?

→ **Yes** → *ADMIT as an 'informal' patient*

↓ **No**

ADMIT using Section 2, 3 or 4

1 Personality disorder characterized by inability to make loving relationships, antisocial behaviour and lack of guilt

135

GP Notes: Sectioning

In practice 'Sectioning' means calling in the duty social worker and duty psychiatrist. It can be a time-consuming and frustrating business. Always try to obtain voluntary admission—it is better for you and the patient.

Keep a supply of forms you might need for Sectioning—Forms 3, 7 and 10 (GP recommendation for Section 2, 4 and 3 respectively) and Form 5 (Application for Section 4 for a 'nearest relative').

Deputizing GPs should always try and contact the patient's own GP.

ⓘ The Mental Health Act only allows for compulsory assessment and treatment of a patient's mental health problems—the patient may refuse consent for investigation and/or treatment of other health problems whilst 'sectioned'.

Sections of the Mental Health Act relevant to GPs: Table 4.1.
In addition:
- *Section 115:* allows an approved social worker to enter and inspect any premises (except hospital) in which a person with a mental disorder is living if s/he has reasonable cause to believe that person is not under proper care. Application through a magistrate is needed.
- *Section 135:* gives right of entry of a police officer who believes a person with a mental disorder is being ill-treated or suffering from self-neglect to enter premises and remove that person to a place of safety. The police officer who attends must be accompanied by an approved social worker and doctor unless the person is already 'sectioned' and absent without leave. Requires application to a magistrate.

Mental Health Community Act (1995): This Act aims to 'provide a system of supervision of care in the community of certain patients who have been detained in hospital'. In England and Wales, the responsible medical officer applies for 'after-care under supervision' (ACUS) to the responsible health authority 6-monthly for the first year then yearly. Application can only be made in respect of a patient ($\geq$16y. old) currently liable to be detained in hospital due to a mental disorder where:
- there could be serious risk of harm to the patient or others if the patient were not to receive further care services *and*
- supervision would help to ensure receipt of further care services.

If patients refuse treatment, they cannot be treated against their will but can be conveyed to a day centre or hospital.

Scotland: The Mental Health Act (Care and Treatment)(Scotland) 2003 provides for compulsory admission under Part 5 for 72h. The application is made by a fully registered medical practitioner in consultation with a mental health officer, unless this is impracticable. In hospital Part 6 (lasting 28d.) can be applied and then, if necessary, Part 7 (Compulsory Treatment Order) for 6mo.

Further information: 🖳 www.scotland.gov.uk

Further reading:
Hyperguide to the Mental Health Act
🖳 www.hyperguide.co.uk/mha

Table 4.1 Sections of the Mental Health Act relevant to general practice

Section	Notes	Application
Section 2: *Admission for assessment:*	Most commonly used section in the community. Admission for 28d. for assessment. Not renewable after that time. Patients may appeal within 2wk. of detention via the Mental Health Tribunal.	Application must be made by the nearest relative or an ASW on the recommendation of 2 doctors—one approved, and the other who has prior knowledge of the patient (☐ p.134). If application is made by the ASW, the nearest relative should be informed before application or as soon as possible afterwards. Application is valid for 14d.
Section 3: *Admission for treatment:*	Admission for treatment for ≤6 mo. The exact mental disorder must be stated. Detention is renewable for a further 6mo. and annually thereafter	Application must be made by the nearest relative or an ASW on the recommendation of 2 doctors—one approved, and the other who has prior knowledge of the patient (☐ p.134). Application is valid for14d.
Section 4: *Emergency admission for assessment:*	Used in situations where admission is urgent and compliance with Section 2 would cause undesirable delay. Admission to hospital for 72h. only. Not renewable. Usually converted to a Section 2 on arrival at hospital.	Application must be made by the nearest relative or an ASW. If application is made by the ASW, the nearest relative should be informed before application or as soon as possible afterwards. Medical recommendation is from *either* an approved doctor or a doctor with prior knowledge of the patient. Application is only valid for 24h.
Section 7: *Guardianship*	A Guardian has power to: • require a person to live at a particular place • require a person to go to specific places at specific times for medical treatment, work, education or training • require a doctor, ASW or other specified person be given access to the person under Guardianship. ❶ Guardians can insist a person sees a doctor but cannot force treatment.	Application must be made by the nearest relative or an ASW on the recommendation of 2 doctors—one approved, and the other who has prior knowledge of the patient (☐ p.134). Application is valid for 14d.

Certifying fitness to work

Own occupation test: Applies for the first 28wk. of their illness to those claiming:
- statutory sick pay from their employer
- incapacity benefit who have done a substantial amount of work in the 21wk. prior to the illness.

The doctor assesses whether the patient is fit to do their *own* job.

Personal capability assessment *(formerly the 'All work test')*: Assesses a patient on a variety of different mental and physical health dimensions for ability to work. Not diagnosis dependent. Applies to:
- everyone after 28wk. incapacity
- those who do not qualify for the own occupation test from the start of their incapacity.

Claimants are sent form IB50 to complete themselves and are asked to obtain form Med4 from their GP. If the Department of Work and Pensions (DWP) is not happy to continue paying their benefit on the basis of these reports, the applicant is called for a medical examination. Conditions relevant to mental health which exempt patients from further examination include:
- Receipt of highest rate care component of disability living allowance (DLA), constant attendance allowance or >80% disabled for other benefit purposes
- Severe mental illness or dementia
- Severe learning disabilities.

Private certificates: Some employers request private certificates in the 1st week of sickness absence. They should request it in writing. if the GP chooses to provide the service, (s)he may charge both for a private consultation and the provision of a private certificate. The company should accept full responsibility for all fees incurred by the patient.

Permitted work: Incapacity benefits do allow very limited work—therapeutic work (must be done as part of a treatment programme and in an institution which provides sheltered work for people with disabilities); voluntary work; local authority councillor; disability expert on an appeal tribunal or member of the Disability Living Allowance advisory board (not >1d./wk.).

Disability Discrimination Act 1995: In some circumstances requires employers to make reasonable adjustments for an employee with a long-term disability. Advise patients to seek specialist advice.

Disability Employment Advisors: Provided by the Employment Service to assist disabled patients to get back to work. Contacted by:
- writing a comment to the effect that intervention would be helpful in the comments box on form Med3 *or*
- writing to the local Jobcentre (with the patient's permission).

Table 4.2 Forms for certifying incapacity to work	
Form	Use
SC1	Self-certification form for people not eligible to claim statutory sick pay who wish to claim incapacity benefit. Certifies first 7d of illness. Available from local Jobcentre Plus offices and GP surgery.
SC2	As SC1 but for people who can claim statutory sick pay. Available from employer, local Jobcentre Plus offices and GP surgery.
Med3	Filled in by GP or hospital doctor who knows the patient for periods of incapacity to work likely to be >7d. If return within 14d. is forecast give fixed date of return ('closed certificate'). If longer, specify a period of time (e.g. 2 mo.) ('open certificate'). Before the patient returns to work reassess and give further certificate with fixed date of return. Only one Med3 can be issued per patient per period of sickness. If mislaid reissue and mark 'duplicate'.
Med4	See personal capability assessment (opposite). Only completed once for any period of incapacity from work.
Med5	Can be used if: • A doctor has not seen the patient but on the basis of a recent (<1mo) written report from another doctor is satisfied that the patient should not work—the certificate should not cover a forward period of >1mo.; • The patient returned to work without receiving a closed certificate (see Med3 above); • >1d since the patient was seen (so Med3 or Med4 cannot be issued) but it is clear the disability is ongoing.
Med6	Used when it is felt that putting a diagnosis on a Med3/Med4 would be harmful either directly to a patient or through their employer knowing their diagnosis. A vague diagnosis is put on the form and a Med6 completed which requests the Department of Works and Pensions (DWP) to send a form to obtain more precise details.
RM7	Sent directly to the DWP to request review of the patient by them sooner than would usually be undertaken.

139

GP Notes: Useful information

Department of Work and Pensions. Medical Evidence for Statutory Sick Pay, Statutory Maternity Pay and Social Security Incapacity Benefit purposes: A guide for registered Medical Practitioners. IB204. April 2000. 🖳 www.dwp.gov.uk/medical/medicalib204/index.asp
Disability Discrimination Act 🖳 www.disability.gov.uk

Consent and decisions

Establishing capacity to make decisions: No-one may make decisions on behalf of a competent adult.

A GP asked to give an opinion on a patient's mental capacity, should:
- Have access to the patient's records and ideally know the patient
- Seek information from friends, relatives and carers
- Examine the patient, assess type and degree of deficit and ability to comply with the specific requirements listed for each situation
- Decide if assessment should be postponed while measures are taken to improve capacity
- Record all the above information.

Even if a doctor thinks a proposed action is in the patient's best interests, he/she must not judge the patient capable if that is not clearly the case. If in doubt, seek a second opinion and/or legal advice.

Consent for medical intervention: Implies willingness of a patient to undergo examination, investigation, or treatment (collectively termed 'procedure' on this page). It may be expressed (i.e. specifically says yes or no/signs a consent form) or implied (i.e. complies with the procedure without ever specifically agreeing to it—use with care). For consent to be valid patients:
- Must be competent to make the decision
- Have received sufficient information to take it and,
- Not be acting under duress.

> ⚠ Under 'common law' touching a patient without valid consent may constitute the civil or criminal offence of battery and if the patient suffers harm as a result of treatment, lack of consent may be a factor in any negligence claim. Never exceed the scope of the authority given by a patient, except in an emergency.

If you are the doctor carrying out a procedure, it is *your responsibility* to discuss it with the patient and seek consent. The task may be delegated but the responsibility *remains* yours.

Consent and mentally incapacitated adults: No-one can give or withhold consent to a procedure on behalf of a mentally incapacitated adult except in Scotland, where a 'tutor-dative' with appropriate authority may make medical decisions on behalf of a patient:
- First assess the patient's capacity to make an informed decision about the procedure.
- If the patient lacks capacity to decide, provided they comply, you may carry out any procedure you judge to be in their best interests unless it has been refused in a valid and applicable advance directive.

If the patient does not comply, you may compulsorily treat only within the safeguards laid down by the Mental Health Act 1983 (📖 pp.134–7).

Advance directives: Statements in which a person makes a decision about medical treatment in case he or she becomes incapable of making that decision later.

- Respect any refusal of treatment given when the patient was competent, provided the decision is clearly applicable to present circumstances, and there is no reason to believe that the patient has altered that decision.
- An advance directive is legally binding if it is clearly established, applicable to the current situation and was made without undue pressure from others.
- The BMA recommends doctors should not withhold 'basic care' (e.g. symptom control) even in the face of a directive which specifies that the patient should receive no treatment.
- Where an advance statement is not available, take patients' known wishes into consideration.

Power of attorney: A power of attorney enables one person (the attorney) to administer the financial affairs of another (the donor). It is created by application through a solicitor. It covers financial matters only.
- *Ordinary power of attorney:* ceases to have effect if the patient (donor) becomes mentally incapable; the donor must understand the nature and effect of what he or she is doing.
- *Enduring power of attorney (EPA):* continues if the donor is mentally incapable, provided it is registered with the Court of Protection. At the time of creating the power of attorney, the donor must understand that the:
  - attorney will be able to assume complete authority over the person's affairs and do anything with the donor's property that the donor could have done;
  - authority will continue if the donor becomes mentally incapable and is irrevocable while the donor remains incapable.

🛈 In Scotland, an ordinary power of attorney signed after January 1991 remains valid even if the donor becomes mentally incapable.

Court of Protection: If a person, by reason of mental disorder, becomes incapable of managing his or her affairs but has not previously signed an EPA, it may be necessary for someone, usually the nearest relative, to apply to the Court of Protection for the appointment of a 'receiver' to do so. The medical practitioner will be asked to complete form CP3. Alternatively, if the patient's affairs are simple (e.g. state pension) direct arrangements can be made with relevant authorities.

Testamentary capacity: Capacity to make a will. Anyone can make a will provided:
- They understand the nature and effect of making a will, extent of property being disposed of and claims others may have on that property
- Decisions are not the result of their condition (e.g. due to a delusion)

🛈 Decisions don't have to seem rational to others, especially if consistent with pre-morbid personality.

Fitness to drive, fly and perform other activities

Fitness to drive

> ⚠ Driving licence holders (or applicants) have a legal duty to inform the DVLA of any disability likely to cause danger to the public if they were to drive.

Driving licence types

- *Group 1:* Ordinary licence for driving a car/motorcycle. Old licences expire at 70th birthday and then must be renewed 3 yearly. Applicants are asked to confirm they have no medical disability. If so, no medical examination is necessary. New photocard licences are automatically renewed 10 yearly until age 70y. Minimum age 17y. (16y. if disabled).
- *Group 2:* enable holders to drive lorries and buses. Min. age 21y. Initially valid until 45th birthday then renewable every 5y. until 65th birthday. >65y. renewable annually. Medical examination is needed to renew Group 2 licences. Applicants must bring form D4 (available from post offices) with them. Examinations take ~ ½ h. A fee may be charged by the GP.

Determining fitness to drive: Patients with any disorder which may cause danger to others if they drove, should be advised not to drive and contact the DVLA. The DVLA gives advice on when they can restart.

Specific guidance regarding psychiatric conditions: Table 4.3.

Further information
DVLA *At a glance guide to the current medical standards of fitness to drive for medical practitioners* available from 🖳 www.dvla.gov.uk
Medical advisers from the DVLA can advise on difficult issues—contact: Drivers Medical Unit, DVLA, Swansea SA99 1TU or *Tel:* 01792 761119

Fitness to fly: Passengers are required to tell the airline at the time of booking about any conditions that might compromise their fitness to fly. The airline's medical officer must then decide whether to carry them or not. *Hazards of flying:*

- Cabin pressure—oxygen levels are lower than at ground level and gas in body cavities expands 30% in flight
- Inactivity and dehydration
- Disruption of routine
- Alcohol consumption
- Stress and excitement.

Table 4.3 DVLA guidance about fitness to drive for patients with mental health problems

Condition	Group 1 licence restrictions	Group 2 licence restrictions
Dementia	Annual review. Stop if posing any danger to the public.	Licence revoked.
Anxiety, depression and other neuroses	Unless severe, continue driving. Stop if severe (especially if suicide at the wheel might be a possibility) or if medication inhibits ability to drive.	Licence revoked if serious acute mental illness. Restored if symptom free and stable for ≥6mo.
Psychosis	Licence revoked. Restored if well and stable for ≥3mo., complaint with treatment and free from adverse drug effects which would impair driving. Specialist report required.	Licence revoked for 3y. Restored if stable and off antipsychotic medication which might affect ability to drive. Specialist report required.
Drug or alcohol misuse or dependency	6mo. off driving (1y. after alcohol or drug-related seizure or detoxification for alcohol, opiate, cocaine or benzodiazepine dependence). DVLA arranges assessment prior to licence restoration.	Licence revoked .1y. (3y. if alcohol dependence or misuse of opiates, cocaine or benzodiazepines; 5y. if alcohol- or drug-related seizure). DVLA arranges assessment prior to licence restoration.

GP Notes: What should I do if a patient continues to drive despite advice to stop?

If the patient <u>does not</u> understand the advice to stop driving: inform the DVLA.

If the patient <u>does</u> understand the advice to stop driving:
- Explain your legal duty to breach confidentiality and inform the DVLA if they do not stop driving.
- If the patient still refuses to stop driving, offer a second medical opinion—on the understanding they stop driving in the interim.
- If the patient still continues driving, consider action such as recruiting next-of-kin to the cause—but beware of breach of confidentiality.
- If all else fails, write to the patient to inform him/her of your intention to inform the DVLA.
- If the patient continues to drive, inform the DVLA and write to the patient to confirm a disclosure has been made.

 Always consider contacting your medical defence body for advice.

Fitness to perform sporting activities: GPs are commonly asked to certify fitness to perform sports. Normally the patient will come with a medical form. If there is a form, request to see it before the medical. If there is no form and you are unsure what to check, telephone the sport's governing body or the event organizer. A fee is payable by the patient.

Many gyms and sports clubs also ask older patients and patients with pre-existing conditions or disabilities to check with their GP before they will sign them on. Assuming that a suitable regime is undertaken most people can participate in some form of sporting activity. Consider the patient's baseline fitness, check BP and medications and recommend a gradual introduction to any new forms of exercise.

Pre-employment certification: It is becoming increasingly common for GPs to be asked about the 'medical' suitability of candidates to perform a job. This is not part of the GP's terms of service and therefore a GP can refuse to give an opinion. In all cases where an opinion is given, a fee can be claimed. Common examples are:
- Ofsted forms for childminders
- Care home staff—proof of 'physical and mental fitness'
- Food handlers—certificates of fitness.

GP Notes: Preventing legal action

⚠ **Remember**, signing a form may result in legal action against you should the patient NOT be fit to undertake an activity.

Where possible include a caveat e.g. 'based on information available in the medical notes the patient appears to be fit to ..., although it is impossible to guarantee this.'

If unsure, consult your local LMC or medical defence organization for advice.

Chapter 5

Benefits available for patients with mental health problems

147

Benefits

⚠ Information in this section is up-to-date at the time of going to press but benefits issues change rapidly.

Millions of pounds of benefits go unclaimed every year. This chapter is a rough guide to the benefits available to enable GPs to point their patients in the right direction. It is not intended as a comprehensive reference.

Table 5.1 Guide to agencies involved in delivering benefits to patients

Agency	Function	Website: www. + suffix	Telephone
Department of Work and Pensions (DWP)	Administers all benefits *except:* Tax credits (Inland Revenue) Statutory Sick Pay (employer) Housing benefit (local authority) Council Tax Benefit (local authorities)	dwp.gov.uk	*Benefits Enquiry Line:* 0800 882200 *Help with form completion:* 0800 441144 *Information for employers and the self-employed:* 0845 7143143
Jobcentre Plus	Helps people of working age to find work and get any benefits they are entitled to	jobcentreplus. gov.uk	Contact local office (list available on website)
Pension Service	Provides services and support for pensioners and people looking into pensions and retirement	thepensionservice. gov.uk	Contact area office (list available on website)
Inland Revenue	Administers tax credits	inlandrevenue. gov.uk	Tax credit enquiry line: 0845 300 3900
Disability and Carers Service	Delivers a range of benefits to disabled people and their carers	disability.gov.uk	Contact local disability benefits office (list available on DWP website)
Appeals Service	Provides an independent tribunal body for hearing appeals	appeals-service. gov.uk	N/A

ℹ 0800 numbers are free; 0845 numbers are charged at local rate.

⚠ Benefit fraud. The DWP provides a freefone number which members of the public can telephone in confidence to give information about benefit fraud. ☎ 0800 85 44 40

Further information for health professionals
Department of Work and Pensions (DWP) 🖳 www.dwp.gov.uk

Further information for patients and carers
Government information and services 🖳 www.direct.gov.uk
Citizens Advice Bureau 🖳 www.adviceguide.org.uk
Age Concern: ☎ 0800 00 99 66 🖳 www.ageconcern.org.uk
Help the Aged: ☎ 0800 800 65 65 🖳 www.helptheaged.org.uk
Counsel and Care ☎ 0845 300 7585 🖳 www.counselandcare.org.uk

Pensions and bereavement benefits

War pensions: For people injured whilst serving in the armed forces and their dependants (if injury caused or hastened death). Administered by the Veterans Agency, MoD. No time limit for claims. *Benefits:*

War disablement pension
- *Basic benefits:* based on percentage disablement
  - If <20% disabled—lump sum
  - If >20% disabled—weekly sum (pension)
- *Other benefits:* Allowances if severely disabled e.g.:
  - War Pensioners mobility supplement—for walking difficulty. Holders can apply for the motability scheme and road tax exemption.
  - Constant attendance allowance—for high levels of care.

Medical treatment: Some services and appliances may be paid for by the Veterans Agency (includes prescription charges, nursing home fees).

War Widows and widowers' pensions
Payable if spouse's death was as a result of service as, in certain circumstances, if spouse received a war pension prior to death.

Further information
Veterans Agency ☎ 0800 169 22 77 🖥 www.veteransagency.mod.uk

Retirement pension: A state retirement pension is payable to women aged ≥60y. and men aged ≥65y.—even if still working. Claim forms should be received automatically—if not request one through the local Jobseeker Plus office. Pensions are taxable.

Basic pension: Flat rate amount—different for single people and married couples. If not enough National Insurance (NI) contributions have been paid amounts may ↓. >80y. higher rate payable which is not dependant on NI contributions.

Increase for dependants: Paid if:
- The claimant's spouse is <60y. and earns under a set amount/does not receive certain other benefits.
- The claimant has children (if claim made before April 2003).

Additional pension: State second pension (replaced SERPS). Based on NI contributions and earnings. Workers can opt out of the additional pension scheme, pay into a private or company scheme instead and pay lower NI.

Graduated pension: Some people may be entitled to a graduated pension. This is based on earnings between 1961 and 1975.

Extra pension: For a person who defers claiming retirement pension for up to 5y. Extra pension is payable when retirement pension is claimed.

❶ If hospitalized, retirement pension is payable for 1y. at full rate. After 12 mo., basic pension is ↓ but additional pension stays the same.

Other benefits for pensioners

- *Pension Credit:* 📖 p.152
- *Free colour TV licence:* All pensioners >75y.
- *Winter fuel payment:* Annual payment to all pensioners >60y.
  Freephone advice service ☎ 0800 22 44 88

Home Responsibilities Protection (HRP): Scheme which protects Basic State Pension for people who don't work or have low income and are caring for someone. 🖥 www.thepensionservice.gov.uk

Christmas bonus: One-off payment made to people receiving a retirement pension or income support a few weeks before Christmas.

Bereavement benefits: Payable to men and women whose spouses have died (co-habitation does not count except in Scotland). Bereavement Payment (BPT) is paid where the late spouse has paid enough NI contributions or their death was caused by their employment. Application should be made as soon as possible after death. If the widow/widower remarries or co-habits, benefits are forfeited. Benefits available:

Bereavement payment: Lump sum payable if spouse was not entitled to full basic retirement pension at the time of death.

Widowed parent's allowance: Paid to widows/widowers with children or if pregnant.

Bereavement allowance: Paid for 52wk. from the date of bereavement for spouses >45y. old, not bringing up children and under retirement age.

Other benefits for widows/widowers

- *Funeral payment:* 📖 p.154
- *War Widows/widowers:* contact Veterans Agency (see opposite).

Cold weather payment: 📖 p.154

Table 5.2 Benefits for people with low income

	Eligibility	How to apply	Benefits gained
Income Support (IS)	• ≥18y (16y, in some circumstances) and <60y. • Low income, <£8000 in savings (£16000 if in residential care) and not in receipt of JSA. • <16h paid work/wk. (and partner <24h/wk.)	Form A1 from local Jobcentre plus office.	*Money:* depends on circumstances. *Other benefits:* housing benefit, community tax benefit, health benefits and social fund payments. Children <5y. and pregnant women—free milk and vitamins. Children >5y.—free school meals and, in some areas, uniform grants. *Christmas bonus:* 📖 p.151
JobSeekers Allowance (JSA)	• ≥19y and <60y (women) or <65y (men). • Unemployed or working <16h/wk. • Capable of and available for work • Have a JobSeekers agreement that contracts the recipient to actively seek work.	Apply by visiting local JobCentre.	*Contributions-based JobSeekers allowance:* can claim for up to 26wk. Age-dependent fixed weekly payment. *Income-based JobSeekers allowance:* allowance dependent on circumstances. Entitles claimants to same benefits as income support (see above). *Hardship payments:* available to people disallowed JSA.
Pension credit	*Guarantee credit:* ≥60y. and income below the 'appropriate amount'. Appropriate amount varies according to circumstances. Capital (excluding value of own home) >£6000 is deemed to count as income at the rate of £1/wk/£500 capital. *Savings credit* ≥65y. and income >savings credit starting point:currently ≥£77.45/wk. for a single person or >£123.80 if one of a couple. Depends on level of income and circumstances.	Apply on form PC1 ☎ 08009991234	*Money:* depends on circumstances *Other benefits:* if receiving guarantee credit: automatically eligible for housing benefit, community tax benefit, and social fund payments.

Working Tax Credit (WTC)	• Age ≥16y, working ≥16 h./wk. and responsible for a child (<16y. or 16–19y. in full time education). • Age ≥16y, working ≥16 h./wk. and has a disability. • Age ≥50y, working ≥16 h./wk. and has started work after ≥6mo. of receiving 1 of certain benefits. • Age ≥25y, and working ≥30 h./wk.	Apply to Inland Revenue ☎ 0845 300 3900 🖥 www.inlandrevenue.gov.uk	**Tax credits**—depends on adding together elements: • Basic element—paid to everyone entitled to WTC • Second adult element • Lone parent element • Working >30h./wk. (can combine both parents if have children). • Disability (if working >16h./wk.) • Severe disability (if working >16h./wk.) • Aged ≥50y. and in receipt of certain benefits before resuming work. • Childcare—up to 70% childcare costs.
Children's Tax Credit (CTC)	• Age ≥16y, and • Responsible for ≥1 child (<16y. or 16–19y. in full time education). • Family income <£50,000 pa.	Apply to Inland Revenue ☎ 0845 300 3900 🖥 www.inlandrevenue.gov.uk	**Tax credits:** • Family element—credit for any family eligible—if there is a child <1y. old in the family. • Child element—credit for each individual child in the family—if the child is disabled/severely disabled.
Health Benefits	**Automatic entitlement:** • Age >60y or <16y (19y if in full time education) • Claiming IS or income-based JSA • Pregnant or within 1y. of childbirth. **By application:** • Low income and • Savings <£8000	If automatic exemption, no need to claim. If not, claim using form HC1 available from pharmacies, GP surgeries and local Jobcentre plus offices.	**Free:** • Prescriptions • NHS dentistry • NHS eye tests and glasses, • NHS wigs and fabric supports • Travel to hospital • Milk anc vitamins for pregnant and breast-feeding women, and children <5y.

Table 5.2 Contd

	Eligibility	How to Apply	Benefits gained
Housing Benefit	Low income, living in rented housing. *Exclusions*: Full-time students without dependants, people in residential care or with savings >£16,000.	Via local authority	Pays rent for up to 60wk. Then need to reapply.
Council Tax Benefit and Second Adult rebate	• **Council tax benefit**: Low income. Exclusions as for housing benefit. • **Second adult rebate**: Payable if someone who lives with you is aged >18y, does not pay rent or council tax and has low income. • **Council tax reduction**: If single occupier or disabled. • **Disregarded occupants**: Certain people including students, carers and children, are not counted in calculating the number of people living at a property.	Via local authority	**Council tax benefit**: pays council tax. **Council tax reductions**: • single occupier—25% discount • all disregarded occupants—5% • disabled—reduction to next lowest council tax band.
The 6 Social Fund payments	• **Crisis loan**—anyone except students and people in residential care can apply. • **Budgeting loan**—for large purchases. Must receive IS, pension credit or income-based JSA. • **Funeral payments**—Must receive low income benefit and be responsible for the funeral. • **Cold weather payments**—average temperature <0°C for ≥7d. Must receive IS, pension credit or income-based JSA and live with a pensioner, child <5y. or disabled person. • **Maternity grant** • **Community care grant**— p.155	Cold weather payments should be automatic. All others claim via local Jobcentre plus offices or ▯ www.dwp. gov.uk	• **Crisis loan**, up to £1000, interest free loan repayable when crisis finished over 78wk. • **Budgeting loan**—as crisis loan • **Funeral expenses**—sum towards cost of funeral—usually does not cover full expenses. • **Cold weather payments**—£8.50/wk.

Table 5.3 Benefits for disability and illness

	Eligibility	How to apply	Amount
Statutory Sick Pay	• Employee age ≥16y. and <65y. • Incapable of work due to sickness or disability. • Earning ≥ NI lower earnings limit. • Unable to work ≥4d and <28wk. (inc. days when would not normally work). • Those ineligible may be eligible for incapacity benefit or maternity allowance.	Notify employer of illness—self-certification first 7d (SC2 📖 p. 139); Med3 after that time 📖 p. 139	£68.20/wk. Some employers have more generous arrangements. Paid through normal pay mechanisms.
Incapacity Benefit	• Not entitled to statutory sick pay (includes self-employed). • Unable to work (Med3 certification until Personal Capability Assessment is applied when GP may be asked for short factual report or Med4 📖 p139). • < pensionable age. • Sufficient NI contributions (unless aged <20y.).	Form SC1 available from GP surgeries, hospitals and local social security offices. If employed and unable to claim SSP on form SP1 supplied by employer.	1–28 weeks—£57.65/wk. 29–52 weeks—£68.20/wk. >52 weeks—£76.45/wk. Plus additions for dependants. A higher rate is payable if <45y. when became unable to work or if over state retirement age
Community Care Grant	Receiving Income Support or income-based Jobseeker's allowance and: • want to re-establish or help the applicant or a family member stay in the community • ease exceptional pressure on the applicant or a family member. • to help with certain travel costs.	Form SF300 from local social security offices or 🖥 www.dwp.gov.uk	Minimum payment £30. No maximum amount
Disabled Facilities Grant	For work essential to help a disabled person live an independent life. Means tested.	Apply via local housing department	Any reasonable application for funds is considered.

CHAPTER 5 Benefits available for patients

Table 5.3 Contd

	Eligibility	How to apply	Amount
Disability Living Allowance (DLA)[1]	• Disability >3mo. and expected to last >6mo. More[2]. • <65y. at time of application Mobility Component: Help needed to get about outdoors • *Higher rate:* unable/virtually unable to walk (age >3y.) • *Lower rate:* help to find way in unfamiliar places (age >5y.) Care Component: Help needed with personal care • *Lower rate:* attention/supervision needed for a significant proportion of the day or unable to prepare a cooked meal. • *Middle rate:* attention/supervision throughout the day or repeated prolonged attention or watching over at night. • *Higher rate:* 24 hour attention/supervision day or terminal illness[2]	☎ 0800 882200 (0800 220674 in Northern Ireland) or Leaflet DS704 available from Post Offices or Using claim packs available at CAB and social security offices or 🖥 www.dwp.gov.uk	Mobility Component: *Higher rate:* £42.30/wk. *Lower rate:* £16.05/ wk. Care Component: *Higher rate:* £60.60/wk. *Middle rate:* £40.55/wk. *Lower rate:* £16.05/wk.
Attandance Allowance (AA)[1]	• Disability >3mo. and expected to last >6mo. More[2]. • Aged ≥65y. • Not permanently in hospital or accommodation funded by the local authority. • Needs attention/supervision—higher rate if 24 hour care required/terminal illness[2].	☎ 0800 882200 (0800 220674 in Northern Ireland) or Leaflet DS704 available from Post Offices or 🖥 www.dwp.gov.uk	*Lower rate:* £40.55 *Higher rate:* £60.60 (for people who need day and night care or are terminally ill)

1 No need to receive help to apply. Not means tested.

2 'terminal illness (not expected to live >6mo.)—claim under Special Rules. Claims are processed much faster and the highest care rate is automatically awarded. GP or hospital specialist fills in form DS1500 to provide clinical information to support application (fee can be claimed).

Carer's allowance	• Aged ≥16y.; and • Spends ≥35h./wk. caring for a person with a disability who is getting AA or constant attendance allowance or middle or higher rate care component of DLA; and • Earning ≤£77.00/wk. After allowable expenses • Not in full-time education	Complete form in leaflet DS700 available from local social security offices or 🖥 www.dwp.gov.uk	£43.15/wk. *Plus additions for dependants.* (🔵 no new claims for dependent children have been accepted since April 2003)
🔵			

• People who need someone's help to get out of the house are entitled to free prescriptions.

• *Severe disablement allowance is still paid to those who applied prior to April 2001.*

Chapter 6

The General Medical Services Contract and mental health

The General Medical Services (GMS) Contract

Although there may be some differences in process in each of the four countries of the UK, the principles of the GMS contract apply to all. A total sum for GMS services is given to each primary care trust (PCO) as part of a bigger unified budget allocation. PCOs are responsible for managing the GMS budget locally.

The contract: Made between an individual practice and a PCO. All the partners of the practice, at least one of whom must be a GP, have to sign the contract. It includes:
- National terms applicable to all practices (the 'practice contract')
- Which services will be provided by that practice i.e.
  - essential
  - additional—if not opted out
  - out-of-hours—if not opted out
  - enhanced—if opted in
- Level of quality of essential and additional services that the practice 'aspires' to
- Support arrangements e.g. IT, premises
- Total financial resources i.e. global sum + quality achievement payments + enhanced services payments + premises + IT + dispensing.

Essential services: All practices must undertake these services. *Include:*
- *Day-to-day medical care of the practice population:* health promotion, management of minor and self-limiting illness and referral to secondary care services and other agencies as appropriate
- *General management of patients who are terminally ill*
- *Chronic disease management.*

Additional services: Services the practice will usually undertake but may 'opt out' of. If the practice opts out, the PCO takes responsibility for providing the service instead. The practice then receives a ↓ global sum payment.

Enhanced services: Commissioned by the PCO and paid for *in addition* to the global sum payment. 3 types:
- *Directed enhanced services:* services under national direction with national specifications and benchmark pricing which all PCOs must commission to cover their relevant population.
- *National enhanced services:* services with national minimum standards and benchmark pricing but not directed (i.e. PCOs do not have to provide these services)
- *Services developed locally* to meet local needs (local enhanced services) e.g. enhanced care of the homeless.

Table 6.1 Payment under the GMS contract

Payment	Explanation
The global sum	Major part of the money paid to practices. Paid monthly and intended to cover practice running costs.
	Includes provision for:
	• Delivery of essential services and additional/out of hours services if not opted out
	• Staff costs
	• Career development
	• Locum reimbursement (e.g. for appraisal, career development, and protected time).
Aspiration payments	Advance payments to allow practices to develop services to achieve higher quality standards.
	Aspiration payments are made monthly alongside global sum payments and amount to ≈60% of the points achieved in the previous year (for 2005/6 this was ≈2004/5 points achieved × £124.60/point × 60% × net size and composition adjustment).
Achievement payments	Payments made for the practice's achieved number of points in the quality and outcomes framework (📖 p.162) as measured at the start of the following year.
	Aspiration payments already received are deducted from the total i.e. payment for actual points less aspiration pay.
Payment for 'extra' services	Paid to practices that provide directed enhanced services, national enhanced services and/or local enhanced services to meet local needs.
Minimum practice income guarantee (MPIG)	Protects those practices that lost out under the redistribution effect of the new resource allocation formula.
	Calculated from the difference between the global sum allocation (GSA) under the new GMS contract and the Global sum equivalent (GSE)—the amount the practice would have earned for providing the same service under the old GMS contract ('The Red Book')
	If GSA < GSE a correction factor (CF) will be applied as long as necessary so that $GSA + CF = GSE$.
Other payments	Payments for premises, IT and dispensing (dispensing practices only)

🔘 The Carr–Hill allocation formula is a GMS resource allocation formula for allocating funds for the global sum and quality payments. The formula takes the practice population and then makes a series of adjustments based on the profile of the local community, taking account of determinants of relative practice workload and costs.

The quality and outcomes framework

The quality and outcomes framework (QoF) was developed specifically for the new GMS contract. Financial incentives are used to encourage high quality care.

The domains: The GMS quality framework is divided into 4 domains (see Table 6.2):

- Clinical
- Organizational
- Additional services
- Patient experience

Indicators: Every domain has a set of 'indicators' which relate to quality standards or guidelines that can be achieved within that domain. The indicators were developed by an expert group based on the best available evidence at the time and will be updated regularly. All data should be obtainable from practice clinical systems and Read codes have been developed to make this easier. Indicators are split into 3 types:

- **Structure:** e.g. is a disease register in place?
- **Process:** e.g. is a particular measure being recorded? Is action being taken where appropriate?
- **Outcome:** e.g. how well is the condition being controlled?

Quality points: All achievement against quality indicators converts to points. Each point has a monetary value.

- **Yes/no indicators:** All points are allocated if the result is +ve and none if –ve.
- **Range of attainment:** For most clinical indicators it is not possible to attain 100% results (even if allowed exceptions are applied) so a range of satisfactory attainment is specified. Minimum standard is 25%. Points are allocated in a linear fashion based on comparison with attainment against a maximum standard e.g. If the maximum % for an indicator is 85%, the minimum 25% and the practice achieves 65%, the practice will receive 40/60 (i.e. 2/3) of the available points.

Reporting on quality: Every year each practice must complete a standard return form recording level of achievement and the evidence for that. In addition there is an annual quality review visit by the PCO. Based on these, the PCO confirms level of achievement funding attained and discusses points the practice will 'aspire' to the following year (p.163). The process is confirmed in writing by the PCO and signed off by the practice. The Commission for healthcare audit and inspection (or equivalents in Scotland/NI) checks quality countrywide.

The quality framework and the Personal Medical Services (PMS) contract: Mechanisms for quality delivery and the quality framework are broadly comparable for GMS and PMS practices. PMS practices can apply for aspiration payments and achievement payments in the same way as GMS practices. However, in order to reflect the local nature of the contracts, standards PMS practices are working to do not have to be the same as those contained in the National Quality Framework. Nevertheless, all standards must be: rigorous; evidence-based; monitored fairly; assessed against criteria agreed between PCOs and providers; and, paid at appropriate and equitable rates.

Table 6.2 Calculation of points for quality framework payments

Components of total points score	Points	Way in which points are calculated
		Achieving pre-set standards in management of:
Clinical indicators	655	• CHD (including left ventricular dysfunction) • Learning disability • Mental health • Atrial fibrillation • Depression • Stroke and TIA • Dementia • Hypertension • COPD • Hypothyroidism • Asthma • Chronic kidney disease • Epilepsy • DM • Cancer • Obesity • Palliative care
Organizational	181	Achieving pre-set standards in: • Records and information about patients • Information for patients • Education and training • Medicines management • Practice management
Additional services	36	Achieving pre-set standards in: • Cervical screening • Child health surveillance • Maternity services • Contraceptive services
Patient experience	108	Achieving pre-set standards in: • Patient survey* • Consultation length
Holistic care	20	Reflects range of achievement across clinical indicators—calculated by ranking clinical indicators in terms of proportion of points gained (1–10). Proportion of the points gained by the 3rd lowest indicator (i.e. indicator ranked 7) is the proportion of the holistic care points obtained.
Total possible	1000	

In 2005/6 and 2006/7 the average value of 1 point = £124.60

*Improving Patient Questionnaire (IPQ—charge payable)—🖳 http://projects.ex.ac.uk/cfep/ipq.htm or General Practice Assessment Questionnaire (GPAQ)—🖳 http://www.gpaq.info

Further information

DoH: The GMS contract. 🖳 http://www.dh.gov.uk
BMA: The Blue book and supporting documents http://www.bma.org.uk

The Mental Health Indicators of the quality and outcomes framework

Maximising points: In 2006/7, 39 points out a total of 1000 are available for mental health quality indicators.

Disease register: Mental Health Indicator 1 requires the practice to 'produce a register of people with schizophrenia, bipolar affective disorder or other psychosis'. The practice reports the number of patients on its mental health disease register as a proportion of total list size.

Regular review: Mental Health Indicator 2 requires practices to review patients with schizophrenia, bipolar affective disorder or other psychosis. The practice reports the percentage of patients on the mental health disease register (above) who have been reviewed within 15 months. The quality target requires the review to include health promotion and prevention advice appropriate to the age, gender and health status of the patient.

In general, reviews should include:

- *A check on the accuracy of prescribed medication:* Review prescribed medication against what patient takes
- *Physical health:* including:
  - regular preventive care, e.g. cervical cytology
  - issues relating to alcohol or drug use
  - smoking and heart disease (including history suggestive of arrhythmias)
  - risk of diabetes from olanzepine and risperidone
- *Co-ordination arrangements with 2° care:* Record details of CPN, Psychiatrist, and other secondary care contacts

ⓘVerification may involve randomly selecting a number of patient case records to ensure review has taken place and been recorded.

Mental Health Indicator 7 requires practices to follow up non-attenders within 14d. of them missing their annual review appointment.

Care plan: People who have chronic severe mental illness require ongoing support from both the formal support services (health and social services) and informal carers - usually other family members. Mental health indicator 6 requires practices to ensure a comprehensive care plan is in place for each patient and that the care plan has been agreed with both the patient and any other individuals involved with the patient's care.

Table 6.3 Mental Health Indicators

Indicator	Description	Points	Payment stages
Records			
Mental Health 1	The practice can produce a register of people with schizophrenia, bipolar affective disorder or other psychosis	4 points	
Ongoing Management			
Mental Health 2	% of patients with schizophrenia, bipolar affective disorder or other psychosis with a review recorded in the preceding 15 mo. This review should include routine health promotion and prevention advice appropriate to the age, gender and health status of the patient	up to 23 points	40–90%
Mental Health 4	% of patients on lithium therapy with a record of serum creatinine and TSH in the preceding 15mo.	up to 1 points	40–90%
Mental Health 5	% of patients on lithium therapy with a record of lithium levels in the therapeutic range within the previous 6mo.	up to 2 points	40–70%
Mental Health 6	% of patients on the register who have a comprehensive care plan documented in the records agreed between individual, their family and/or carers as appropriate	up to 6 points	25–50%
Mental Health 7	% of patients with schizophrenia, bipolar affective disorder and other psychosis, who do not attend the practice for their annual review, who are identified and followed up by practice team within 14d. of non attendance.	up to 3 points	40–90%

Note: Previous Mental Health 3 was removed in the updated Quality and Outcomes Framework (2006)

CHAPTER 6 **GMS Contract & Mental health**

Monitoring lithium therapy: Mental Health Indicators 4 and 5 are all concerned with monitoring of lithium therapy. Lithium salts are used in the prophylaxis and treatment of mania, in the prophylaxis of bipolar disorder (manic-depressive disorder) and in the prophylaxis of recurrent depression (unipolar illness or unipolar depression). The decision to give prophylactic lithium requires specialist advice.

Monitoring lithium levels: Mental Health Indicator 5 requires practices to check serum lithium levels. The practice reports the percentage with levels in the therapeutic range in the previous 6mo. (Indicator 5).

Lithium salts have a narrow therapeutic index (therapeutic:toxic ratio). Intercurrent illness, declining renal function or co-prescription of other drugs which reduce lithium excretion (e.g. thiazide diuretics or NSAIDs) can result in toxicity. Serum monitoring with a blood sample taken 12h. after the preceding dose is essential.

Doses are adjusted to achieve serum lithium concentration of 0.6–1mmol/l. If the range differs locally the PCO is required to allow for this. Levels <0.6 may be acceptable, depending on clinical circumstances. For this reason, the top standard for this indicator is set lower, at 70%. Levels >1.5mmol/l may be fatal.

Monitoring serum creatinine and TSH: In long-term use lithium has been associated with hypothyroidism (8–15%), hypercalcaemia and abnormal renal function. Mental Health Indicator 4 requires practices to check serum creatinine and TSH in all patients on lithium. The practice reports the percentage of patients who have had these checks in the preceding 15mo.

Creating a system for lithium monitoring: Where a practice is prescribing the lithium, it has responsibility for checking that routine blood tests have been done (not necessarily by the practice) and for following up defaulters.
- Compile a list of all those on lithium treatment
- Record the date of the last lithium test and create a call-recall system to ensure patients are called for testing.
- Ensure someone is responsible for chasing up defaulters, checking results as they come in, acting on abnormal results and ensuing results are recorded on computer

ⓘVerification may involve inspecting the computer output and/or randomly selecting a number of patient records to ensure lithium, TSH and creatinine levels have been checked.

GP Notes: Lithium cards

A lithium treatment card available from pharmacies tells patients:
- How to take lithium preparations
- What to do if a dose is missed, *and*
- What side-effects to expect.

It also explains why regular blood tests are important and warns that some medicines and illnesses can change serum-lithium concentration.

Cards may be obtained from NPA Services, 38–42 St. Peter's St, St. Albans, Herts AL1 3NP.

Dementia, depression and learning disability indicators

These indicators have been newly introduced from 1st April 2006.

Dementia indicators: Dementia is common and patients with dementia require a great deal of support from both their carers and the health and social care services. The new dementia indicators aim to identify patients with dementia and ensure adequate support is in place for both patients and their carers.

Dementia register: Dementia 1 requires practices to create a register of patients with dementia. The practice reports the number of patients on its dementia register as a proportion of total list size.

Annual review: Dementia 2 requires practices to review the care of dementia patients annually. Reviews should focus on support needs of the patient and their carer and address 3 key issues:
- The carers' needs for information commensurate with the stage of the illness and their and the patients' health and social care needs
- The impact of caring on the care-giver
- Communication and co-ordination arrangements with secondary care.

Depression indicators: Depression is common and under-diagnosed—particularly amongst patients with chronic disease. The new depression indicators aim to screen for depression in high risk groups and ensure objective measurements of severity are obtained early after diagnosis so that management can be tailored to severity and progress can be measured objectively.

Screening for depression: Depression 1 requires practices to screen patients on the coronary heart disease and diabetes registers for depression with at least 2 standard screening questions:
- During the last month, have you often been bothered by feeling down, depressed or hopeless?
- During the last month, have you often been bothered by having little interest or pleasure in doing things?

Patients replying yes to either question require further mood assessment.

Assessing severity: For those patients with a new diagnosis of depression in the last 12 months, depression 2 requires practices to perform an assessment of severity at the outset of treatment using an assessment tool validated for use in primary care. The 3 suggested severity measures validated for use in a primary care setting are the Patient Health Questionnaire (PHQ-9—📖 p.6), the Beck Depression Inventory Second Edition (BDI-II) and the Hospital Anxiety and Depression Scale (HADS).

Learning disability register: Learning disability 1 requires practices to compile a register of patients with learning disability. Learning disability is not defined, so know your criteria for inclusion and be prepared to justify them.

Table 6.4 Dementia, depression and learning disability indicators

Indicator	Description	Points	Payment stages
Dementia			
Dementia 1	The practice can produce a register of patients diagnosed with dementia	5 points	
Dementia 2	% of patients diagnosed with dementia whose care has been reviewed in the preceding 15mo. This should include an assessment of support needs of the patient and their carer and a review of co-ordination arrangements with secondary care	up to 15 points	25–60%
Depression			
Depression 1	% of patients with on the coronary heart disease and/or diabetes register for whom case finding for depression has been undertaken on one occasion in the preceding 15mo. using 2 standard screening questions.	up to 8 points	40–90%
Depression 2	For those patients with a new diagnosis of depression in the previous 12mo., the % of patients with an assessment of severity, using an assessment tool validated for use in primary care, recorded in the patient record at the start of treatment	up to 25 points	40–90%
Learning disability			
Learning disability 1	The practice can produce a register of patients with learning disabilities	4 points	

Other relevant quality indicators

Medication: For patients with mental illness it is important that:
- The notes have a clear indication of when drugs were started and what they were prescribed for (Records Indicator 9)
- Regular review of repeat medication is carried out - even for those not deemed to have severe enough mental illness to be on the mental health register (Medicines Indicator 9)
- When the practice has a responsibility for administering medication (e.g. regular neuroleptics) there is a call-recall system to make sure patients don't slip through the net (Medicines Indicator 7)

Carers: Many patients with chronic mental health problems are looked after by informal carers (📖 p.130). As a result of their caring role, many carers develop physical and mental health problems. Indentifying and supporting them (Management Indicator 9) can help maintain carer health and keep patients in the community longer.

Significant event audit (critical event monitoring): Recognised methodology for reflecting on important events in a practice. Practices undertaking significant event audit are eligible for quality points (Education Indicators 2 & 7). Discussion of specific events can:
- Identify learning objectives *and*
- Provoke emotions that can be harnessed to achieve change.

For it to be effective, it must be practised in a culture that avoids blame and involves all disciplines. 3 steps:
- *Decide on a topic and plan a meeting.* A list of suitable events can be made for an individual practice or a pre-formed list of suitable events is available from the RCGP (Significant Event Auditing: Occasional Paper 70, 1995). Suitable mental health events include suicide and/or Section under the Mental Health Act.
- At the end of the discussion, *come to a decision* about the case e.g. well managed, need change in procedure etc.
- *Prepare a report.* The 2 acceptable formats for laying out these reports are described in table 6.4.

Table 6.4 **Methods of reporting significant event audits**	
Reporting Method 1	**Reporting Method 2**
Description of event—This should be brief and can be in note form.	*What happened?*
Learning outcome—This should describe the aspects which were of high standard and those which could be improved. Where appropriate it should include why the event occurred.	*Why did it happen?* *Was insight demonstrated?* *Was change implemented?*
Action plan—The decision(s) taken need to be contained in the report. The reasons for these decisions should be described together with any other lessons learned from the discussion.	

Table 6.5 Other relevant indicators

Indicator	Description	Points	Payment stages
Records 9	For repeat medicines, an indication for the drug can be identified in the records (for drugs added to the repeat prescription with effect from 1 April 2004)	4 points	Minimum standard 80%
Education 2	The practice has undertaken a minimum of three significant event reviews in the past year	6 points	For 3 reviews
Education 7	The practice has undertaken a minimum of twelve significant event reviews in the past 3 years which could include: • Any death occurring in the practice premises • New cancer diagnoses • Deaths where terminal care has taken place at home • Any suicides • Sections under the Mental Health Act • Child protection cases • Medication errors • A significant event occurring when a patient may have been subjected to harm had the circumstances/outcome been different (near miss)	4 points	For 12 reviews
Management 9	The practice has a protocol for the identification of carers and a mechanism for the referral of carers for social services assessment	3 points	
Medicines 7	Where the practice has responsibility for administering regular injectable neuroleptic medication, there is a system to identify and follow up patients who do not attend	4 points	
Medicines 9	A medication review is recorded in the notes in the preceding 15 months for all patients being prescribed repeat medicines	8 points	Minimum standard 80%

National enhanced services

These are services with national minimum standards and benchmark pricing but are not 'directed' (i.e. PCTs do not have to provide these services).

Specialized care of patients with depression

Practices performing this service must:
- Maintain a register of depressed patients
- Use screening questionnaires/interviews to improve detection of depression
- Apply a multidisciplinary approach to management of depression using drug treatment and non-drug treatment and referring on to other services where appropriate
- Produce and maintain a personal health plan for each patient
- Review the service annually including
  - audit of the register of patients
  - audit of antidepressant medication use and effect on treatment outcomes.
  - obtaining feedback from patients and their families using the standardized patient satisfaction questionnaire.

€ *Funding available: £1000/year + annual payment in arrears of £80–£100/patient.*

Patients who are alcohol misusers

To provide this service practices must:
- Develop a register of all patients who admit they are alcohol misusers
- Undertake brief interventions and offer support to carry out behavioural change
- Arrange follow-up treatment which might include counselling in conjunction with local alcohol services, or referral to a day programme or alcohol rehabilitation centre
- Provide detoxification in the community or home setting
- Routinely use alcoholism assessment tools
- Liaise with local specialist alcohol treatment services
- Provide or arrange training for any team members involved
- Carry out an annual review of the service including audit.

€ *Funding available: £1000/year + £200/patient/year quarterly in arrears.*

Patients suffering from drug misuse

Before applying to provide this service the following must be in place:
- An accurate register of patients
- Sequential review as appropriate
- Safe and secure premises appropriate for provision of such services
- A good knowledge and effective liaison with local drug services and other relevant agencies
- Links between local pharmacies, primary care drug support workers, social services and local mental and clinical health teams.

This service will fund practices to:
- Develop and co-ordinate the care of local drug users
- Develop practice guidelines (including incorporating local drug detoxification procedures and national guidelines on treatment of drug misuse)
- Treat dependent drug users with support (e.g. from specialist drug rehabilitation services)—this includes prescription of substitute drugs and antagonists
- Address co-existing problems of drug users including co-existing physical, emotional, social and legal problems
- Act as a resource for other practitioners
- Provide additional training and continuing professional development for clinicians involved in the scheme and other support staff
- Maintain the safety of staff
- Review the service by participating in audit of prescribing practice and hepatitis B screening and immunization data every 6 months and annual review of attendance rate, outcomes and costs.

€ *Funding available: £1000/year + £500 withdrawal/patient/year + £350 maintenance/patient/year, paid quarterly in arrears.*

Chapter 7

Useful information and contacts

Useful information and contacts for GPs

General information

Centre for Evidence Based Mental Health. Includes information on research, education, workshops, and links to other sites.
🖳 www.cebmh.com

DIPEx patient experience database 🖳 www.dipex.org

Hyperguide to the Mental Health Act 🖳 www.hyperguide.co.uk/mha

The Mental Health Act (Care and Treatment)(Scotland) 2003
🖳 www.scotland.gov.uk

WHO Guide to Mental and Neurological Health in Primary Care.

Includes guidelines, patient resources, and checklist questionnaires.
🖳 www.mentalneurologicalprimarycare.org

Addiction and dependence

BMJ *Addiction and dependence—II: alcohol.* (1997) 315, 358–360.
🖳 www.bmj.com

DoH Drug misuse and dependence—guidelines on clinical management (1999) 🖳 www.dh.gov.uk

DTB Managing the heavy drinker in primary care. (2000) 38(8), 60–64.

SIGN The management of harmful drinking and alcohol dependence in primary care. (2003) 🖳 www.sign.ac.uk

Substance Misuse Management in General Practice (SMMGP)
🖳 www.smmgp.demon.co.uk/index.htm

Anxiety

NICE Management of anxiety (panic disorder, with or without agoraphobia, and generalized anxiety disorder) in adults in primary, secondary and community care (2004) 🖳 www.nice.org.uk

Child protection

DoH 🖳 www.dh.gov.uk
- *Working together to safeguard children* (1998)
- *What to do if you're worried a child is being abused* (2003)

RCGP Carter & Bannon. The role of primary care in the protection of children from abuse and neglect (2003) 🖳 www.rcgp.org.uk

Department for Education and skills *Every Child Matters* (2004)
🖳 www.everychildmatters.gov.uk

Chronic fatigue syndrome

Kings College 🖳 www.kcl.ac.uk/cfs

Royal Australian College of Physicians *Chronic Fatigue Syndrome*
🖳 www.mja.com.au/public/guides/cfs/cfs1.html

Counselling

Bower *et al.* The clinical effectiveness of counselling in primary care (2003) *Psychol Med* 33: 203–15.

Depression

Mild depression in general practice (2003) *DTB* 4(8) 60–4.
NICE Management of depression in primary and secondary care (2004)
🖳 www.nice.org.uk

Disability and benefits

Department of Work and Pensions (DWP) 🖳 www.dwp.gov.uk

DWP *Medical Evidence for Statutory Sick Pay, Statutory
Maternity Pay and Social Security Incapacity Benefit purposes:
A guide for registered Medical Practitioners.* IB204. April 2000.
🖳 www.dwp.gov.uk/medical/medicalib204/index.asp

Disability Discrimination Act 🖳 www.disability.gov.uk

DVLA *At a glance guide to the current medical standards of fitness to
drive for medical practitioners* available from 🖳 www.dvla.gov.uk

Medical advisers from the DVLA can advise on difficult issues—contact:
Drivers Medical Unit, DVLA, Swansea SA99 1TU or ☎ 01792 761119

Health and Safety Executive (HSE) 🖳 www.hse.gov.uk/stress

Jobcentre Plus 🖳 jobcentreplus.gov.uk

Eating disorders

NICE *Core interventions in the treatment and management of anorexia
nervosa, bulimia nervosa and related eating disorders* (2004)
🖳 www.nice.org

GP contract

DoH: *The GMS Contract* 🖳 www.dh.gov.uk

BMA: The Blue book and supporting documents 🖳 www.bma.org.uk

Post-traumatic stress disorder

NICE *Post-traumatic stress disorder (PTSD): the management of PTSD in
adults and children in primary, secondary and community care* (2005)
🖳 www.nice.org.uk

Suicide and self-harm

DoH National Suicide Prevention Strategy for England (2002)
🖳 www.dh.gov.uk

NICE Self-harm: The short-term physical and psychological management and secondary prevention of self-harm in primary and secondary
care (2004). 🖳 www.nice.org.uk

Information and contacts for patients, relatives and carers

National Association for Mental Health (MIND) ☎ 020 8519 2122
🖳 www.mind.org.uk

Royal College of Psychiatrists: Patient information sheets
🖳 www.rcpsych.ac.uk

DIPEx patient experience database 🖳 www.dipex.org

Addiction and dependence

ADFAM Support for families of addicts. ☎ 020 7928 8898
🖳 www.adfam.org.uk

Alcoholics Anonymous ☎ 0845 7697555
🖳 www.alcoholics-anonymous.org.uk

Alcohol Concern 🖳 www.alcoholconcern.org.uk

Benzodiazepines 🖳 www.benzo.org.uk

Drinkline (government-sponsored helpline) ☎ 0800 917 8282

Drugs-info Information about substance abuse for families of addicts
🖳 www.drugs-info.co.uk

Drugscope Information about drug abuse and how to get treatment
🖳 www.drugscope.org.uk

Ecstasy 🖳 www.ecstasy.org

'Know the Score' (Scotland) ☎ 0800 587 5879
🖳 www.knowthescore.info

National Treatment Agency for Substance Abuse 🖳 www.nhs.uk

Solvent abuse ☎ 0808 800 2345 🖳 www.re-solv.org

'Talk to FRANK' (England and Wales) Government-run information,
advice and referral service. ☎ (24 hour) 0800 77 66 00
🖳 www.talktofrank.com

ADHD

Green & Chee *Understanding ADHD* (1997) Vermilion ISBN
0091817005

National attention deficit disorder information and support service
(ADDISS) ☎ 020 8906 9068 🖳 www.addiss.co.uk

Autism

National autistic society of the UK (NAS) ☎ 0845 070 4004
🖳 www.nas.org.uk

Benefits

Benefit fraud line ☎ 0800 85 44 40

Citizens Advice Bureau 🖳 www.adviceguide.org.uk

Department of Work and Pensions 🖳 www.dwp.gov.uk
☎ *Benefits Enquiry Line*—0800 882200; 0800 243355 (minicom facility);
0800 441144 (for help with form completion).

Government information and services 🖳 www.direct.gov.uk

Inland Revenue 🖳 www.inlandrevenue.gov.uk Tax credit enquiry line
☎ 0845 300 3900

Jobcentre Plus 🖳 www.jobcentreplus.gov.uk

Pension Service 🖳 www.thepensionservice.gov.uk

Veterans Agency ☎ 0800 169 22 77 🖳 www.veteransagency.mod.uk

Bereavement

CRUSE ☎ 0870 167 1677 🖳 www.crusebereavementcare.org.uk

National Association of Widows ☎ 024 7663 4848
🖳 www.widows.uk.net

Bipolar disorder

Manic Depression Fellowship ☎ 020 8974 6550 🖳 www.mdf.org.uk

Carers

Carers UK ☎ 0808 808 7777 🖳 www.carersonline.org.uk

Counsel and Care ☎ 0845 300 7585 🖳 www.counselandcare.org.uk

Princess Royal Trust for Carers ☎ 020 7480 7788 🖳 www.carers.org

Disability and Carers Service 🖳 www.disability.gov.uk

Childhood behaviour problems

Cry-sis Support for families with crying and sleepless babies
☎ 020 7404 5011 🖳 www.cry-sis.com

Green *Beyond Toddlerdom: Every Parent's Guide to the 5–10s* (2000)
Vermilion ISBN 0091816246

Green *Toddler taming: A parents guide to the first four years* (2000)
Vermilion ISBN 0091875285

Parentline ☎ 0808 800 2222 🖳 www.parentlineplus.org.uk

179

Child abuse

Childline 24h. confidential counselling service ☎ 0800 1111
🖳 www.childline.org

Chronic fatigue syndrome

Action for ME ☎ 0845 123 2380 🖳 www.afme.org.uk

ME Association ☎ 0870 444 1836 🖳 www.meassociation.org.uk

Dementia
Alzheimer's Society ☎ 0845 300 0336 🖳 www.alzheimers.org.uk

Dementia Care Trust ☎ 0870 443 5325 🖳 www.dct.org.uk

Depression
Depression Alliance ☎ 020 7207 3293 🖳 www.depressionalliance.org

Dyslexia
British Dyslexia Association ☎ 0118 966 8271
🖳 www.bda-dyslexia.org.uk

Dyspraxia
Dyspraxia Foundation: ☎ 01462 454 986
🖳 www.dyspraxiafoundation.org.uk

Eating Disorders
Eating Disorders Association (EDA) ☎ 0845 634 1414 (Adults)
0845 634 7650 (Youths) 🖳 www.edauk.com

Elderly
Age Concern: ☎ 0800 00 99 66 🖳 www.ageconcern.org.uk

Help the Aged: ☎ 0800 800 65 65 🖳 www.helptheaged.org.uk

Action on Elder Abuse ☎ 0808 808 8141 🖳 www.elderabuse.org.uk

Enuresis
ERIC (enuresis resource and information) 🖳 www.eric .org.uk

Obsessive-compulsive disorder
OCD Action ☎ 020 7226 4000 🖳 www.ocdaction.org.uk

Panic disorder
No More Panic 🖳 www.nomorepanic.co.uk

Personality disorder
Borderline UK 🖳 www.borderlineuk.co.uk

Borderline Personality Disorder (BPD) Central 🖳 www.bpdcentral.com

Phobias
Triumph Over Phobia (TOP) UK. Self-help materials and groups
☎ 01225 330 353 🖳 www.triumphoverphobia.com

Postnatal depression
National Childbirth Trust (NCT) ☎ 0870 770 3236 Info line
0870 444 8707 🖳 www.nctpregnancyandbabycare.com

Schizophrenia
Rethink (National Schizophrenia Fellowship) ☎ 020 8974 6814
🖳 www.nsf.org.uk

Severe learning difficulty

MENCAP ☎ 0808 808 1111 🖳 www.mencap.org.uk

Sexual health

Brook Advisory Service Contraceptive advice and counselling for teenagers. ☎ 0800 0185 023 🖳 www.brook.org.uk

Sexwise for under 19s ☎ 0800 28 29 30

Special education

Independent Panel for Special Education Advice (IPSEA)
☎ 0800 018 4016 (Scotland—0131 665 4396; Northern Ireland—0232 705654) 🖳 www.ipsea.org.uk

Children of High Intelligence 🖳 www.chi-charity.org.uk

Stress

International Stress Management Association (UK) ☎ 07000 780 430
🖳 www.isma.org.uk

Stress Management Society ☎ 0870 199 3260 🖳 www.stress.org.uk

Suicide and self-harm

Samaritans 24h. emotional support via telephone ☎ 08457 909 090

Self Injury and Related Issues (SIARI) 🖳 www.siari.co.uk

Survivors of Bereavement by Suicide ☎ 0870 241 3337
🖳 www.uk-sobs.org.uk

Index

183